Clinical
Examina...

Pete ...ledge BSc MBChB MRCPCH PCME MSc
Con... ...Paediatrician
Le... ...eral Infirmary
L...

...artledge BSc MBChB DRCOG FSRH
...ainee in General Practice
...d Humber Deanery

...key MBChB MMedEd DA(UK)
...MC FCEM FERC
...n Emergency Medicine
...Medical Education
...and Huddersfield Foundation Trust

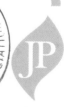

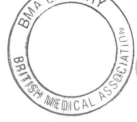

JP
medical
publishers

BRITISH MEDICAL ASSOCIATION

0780569

© 2014 JP Medical Ltd.

Published by JP Medical Ltd, 83 Victoria Street, London, SW1H 0HW, UK

Tel: +44 (0)20 3170 8910

Fax: +44 (0)20 3008 6180

Email: info@jpmedpub.com

Web: www.jpmedpub.com

The rights of Peter Cartledge, Catherine Cartledge and Andrew Lockey to be identified as the authors of this work have been asserted by them in accordance with the Copyright, Designs and Patents Act 1988.

All rights reserved. No part of this publication may be reproduced, stored or transmitted in any form or by any means, electronic, mechanical, photocopying, recording or otherwise, except as permitted by the UK Copyright, Designs and Patents Act 1988, without the prior permission in writing of the publishers. Permissions may be sought directly from JP Medical Ltd at the address printed above.

All brand names and product names used in this book are trade names, service marks, trademarks or registered trademarks of their respective owners. The publisher is not associated with any product or vendor mentioned in this book.

Medical knowledge and practice change constantly. This book is designed to provide accurate, authoritative information about the subject matter in question. However readers are advised to check the most current information available on procedures included and check information from the manufacturer of each product to be administered, to verify the recommended dose, formula, method and duration of administration, adverse effects and contraindications. It is the responsibility of the practitioner to take all appropriate safety precautions. Neither the publisher nor the authors assume any liability for any injury and/or damage to persons or property arising from or related to use of material in this book.

This book is sold on the understanding that the publisher is not engaged in providing professional medical services. If such advice or services are required, the services of a competent medical professional should be sought.

ISBN: 978-1-907816-75-8

British Library Cataloguing in Publication Data
A catalogue record for this book is available from the British Library

Library of Congress Cataloging in Publication Data
A catalog record for this book is available from the Library of Congress

JP Medical Ltd is a subsidiary of Jaypee Brothers Medical Publishers (P) Ltd, New Delhi, India.

Publisher:	Richard Furn
Development Editors:	Thomas Fletcher, Paul Mayhew
Editorial Assistant:	Sophie Woolven
Design:	Designers Collective Ltd

Typeset, printed and bound in India.

Preface

Proficiency in history-taking and clinical examination is fundamental to good clinical practice. To acquire it, you will require practical skills and a thorough understanding of the systems of the body. You will also need to be able to work in partnership with your patients, listening to their concerns and respecting their individuality and dignity.

Pocket Tutor Clinical Examination helps you develop this wide range of skills. The first two chapters outline the general principles of structuring a consultation, taking a history and conducting an examination. Approaches to forming a differential diagnosis and following up a consultation are included, along with ethicolegal considerations and a summary of the relevance of evidence-based medicine to clinical skills.

Ten systems-based chapters then follow, each one starting with a recap of key anatomy and physiology before describing system-specific symptoms and signs. Subsequent discussion of clinical examination guides you through the most commonly used techniques. Each systems chapter closes with a summary of common investigations likely to be requested as a result of positive examination findings, along with a summary table.

Some patient groups require special approaches to history and examination, for example because of communication difficulties or age-related characteristics. Accordingly we devote the final three chapters to children, the elderly and critically ill patients.

We hope this book helps you develop the skills you will need to be a first class clinician.

Peter Cartledge
Catherine Cartledge
Andrew Lockey
March 2014

Acknowledgements

We would like to thank the tireless work of our medical student reviewer Caleb Van Essen whose contribution has been invaluable.

We would also like to thank the following for their specialist contributions:

Dr Caroline Fraser (Cardiovascular system)
Dr Jack Gormley (Cranial nerves)
Mr Edward Hannon (Gastrointestinal system)
Dr Bernice Knight (Psychiatry)
Dr Daniel Langer (Respiratory system)
Dr Natalie McCall (Paediatrics)
Dr Pallai Rappai Shillo (Endocrine system)
Dr Amanda Robinson (Elderly patients)
Dr Kristina Tocce (Female reproductive system)
Mr Sam Vollans (Musculoskeletal system)
Dr Timothy Walker (Neurological system)
Dr Sam Wallis (Medical ethics)
Dr Timothy White (General principles of examination)
Dr Calvin Wilson (Global health)

Figures 2.4b, 2.6b, 2.7b, 2.8, 3.3, 3.7, 5.2a–b, 5.3, 6.1, 7.2, 7.7, 8.3, 9.3, 9.8, 10.6a–c, 10.7a–c, 10.8a–b, 10.9a–c, 10.10a–c, 10.12a–b, 10.13, 10.14a–e, 10.15a–b and 12.1 are reproduced from: Tunstall R, Shah N. Pocket Tutor Surface Anatomy. London: JP Medical, 2012.

Figures 8.2, 8.4 and 9.1 are reproduced from: Goodfellow JA. Pocket Tutor Neurological Examination. London: JP Medical, 2012.

Figure 3.1 is reproduced from: James S, Nelson K. Pocket Tutor ECG Interpretation. London: JP Medical, 2011.

Figure 1.1 is reproduced from: Brugha R, Marlais M, Abrahamson E. Pocket Tutor Paediatric Clinical Examination. London: JP Medical, 2013.

Figure 9.10 is reproduced from: Bhattacharyya A, Patel N. Pocket Tutor Otolaryngology. London: JP Medical, 2012.

Figure 7.3 is reproduced from: Crosbie EJ, et al. Key Clinical Topics in Obstetrics and Gynaecology. London: JP Medical, 2014.

Contents

Preface   *iii*
Acknowledgements   *vi*

Chapter 1 First principles
1.1   The consultation   1
1.2   General principles of history taking   3
1.3   Forming a differential diagnosis   17
1.4   After the consultation   19
1.5   Evidence-based medicine   20
1.6   Ethicolegal considerations   22

Chapter 2 General principles of examination
2.1   General structure of examination   27
2.2   Preparation for the examination   28
2.3   Vital signs (observations)   29
2.4   Techniques for examination   35
2.5   General inspection   37
2.6   The hands   41
2.7   The neck   45
2.8   The face and mouth   48
2.9   Ear, nose and throat   49
2.10 The legs and feet   52
2.11 The skin and hair   52
2.12 Systems examination   53

Chapter 3 Cardiovascular system
3.1   System overview   57
3.2   Symptoms and signs   60
3.3   Examination of the cardiovascular system   65
3.4   Examination of the peripheral vascular system   79
3.5   Common investigations   82
3.6   System summary   82

Chapter 4 Respiratory system
4.1 System overview 85
4.2 Symptoms and signs 87
4.3 Examination of the respiratory system 93
4.4 Common investigations 101
4.5 System summary 102

Chapter 5 Gastrointestinal system
5.1 System overview 103
5.2 Symptoms and signs 106
5.3 Examination of the gastrointestinal system 112
5.4 Common investigations 125
5.5 System summary 126

Chapter 6 Genitourinary system
6.1 System overview 127
6.2 Symptoms and signs 128
6.3 Examination of the genitalia 131
6.4 Common investigations 135
6.5 System summary 135

Chapter 7 Female reproductive system
7.1 System overview 137
7.2 The breast consultation 139
7.3 Examination of the breast 142
7.4 The gynaecological consultation 145
7.5 The gynaecological examination 147
7.6 The obstetric consultation 152
7.7 The obstetric examination 152
7.8 Common investigations 157
7.9 System summary 157

Chapter 8 Neurological system
8.1 System overview 159
8.2 Symptoms and signs 162
8.3 Neurological examination 166
8.4 Examination of the peripheral nervous system 168
8.5 Higher mental function 191
8.6 Common investigations 194
8.7 System Summary 195

Chapter 9 Cranial nerves and ophthalmology

9.1 System overview   197
9.2 Symptoms and signs   199
9.3 Examination of the cranial nerves   202
9.4 Examination of the visual system   214
9.5 Common investigations   216
9.6 System summary   217

Chapter 10 Musculoskeletal system

10.1 System overview   219
10.2 Symptoms and signs   219
10.3 Examination of the musculoskeletal system   223
10.4 Common investigations   243
10.5 System summary   248

Chapter 11 Psychiatry

11.1 Symptoms and signs   249
11.2 The psychiatric assessment   251
11.3 Higher mental function   259
11.4 Common investigations   259
11.5 System summary   260

Chapter 12 Endocrine system

12.1 System overview   261
12.2 Symptoms and signs   262
12.3 Examination of the thyroid   267
12.4 Diabetes   270
12.5 Common investigations   272
12.6 System summary   273

Chapter 13 Paediatrics

13.1 Overview   275
13.2 Symptoms and signs   277
13.3 Examining a child   282
13.4 Development assessment   286
13.5 Examination of the newborn baby   289
13.6 Assessment of child mistreatment   292

Chapter 14 Elderly patients

14.1 Overview   293
14.2 Symptoms and signs   294

14.3 Examination 297
14.4 System summary 302

Chapter 15 Critically ill patients

15.1 Primary survey 305
15.2 Secondary survey 310
15.3 Early warning score systems 311
15.4 Adult advanced life support 311

Index *315*

First principles

1.1 The consultation

Most consultations between a clinician and a patient will follow a very structured pattern: an introduction is followed by a thorough history, which explores the patient's ideas, concerns and expectations. The patient is examined and a differential diagnosis formulated. Investigations are then organised, when necessary, and a treatment plan is put in place. It is said that over 80% of diagnoses in general medical clinics are based on the medical history. So it is of paramount importance to focus time and energy on becoming a good history taker.

At the beginning

Taking a history is not only the key to clinical diagnosis but also the start of the 'doctor–patient' relationship. Every consultation should start the same way:

- Wash your hands
- If working in a clinic (e.g. outpatients or family practice), always come to the door to greet the patient. Never greet a patient sitting down
- Introduce yourself and your role and designation (in lay terms)
- Find out who the patient is (biographical details): the mnemonic **DNA SORAN (Table 1.1)** can be used. These elements don't all have to be taken immediately (a name and age are a minimum), but it is appropriate to take them during the social history. You may ask the patient how he or she wishes to be addressed

Open and closed questions

Doctors will generally interrupt their patients after 18 seconds. This may be necessary in order

> **Clinical insight**
>
> The cornerstones of good clinical practice are taking a thorough history and remaining inquisitive. Remember: listen to the patient, he or she is telling you the diagnosis.

to guide the consultation, but usually it is out of impatience and can significantly reduce the chances of identifying the correct diagnosis. This is difficult because, if allowed to, some patients will continue talking for excessive periods with too much detail.

General: **DNA** **SORAN**	D – date N – name A – age	S – sex O – occupation R – religion A – address N – next of kin
Presenting complaint	List each presenting problem	
History of presenting complaint	Use the OPERATES+ mnemonic for each presenting problem (**Table 1.2**) Use the SOCRATES mnemonic for pain history (**Table 1.3**)	
Past medical history **Past surgical history**	Previous illnesses or surgery Important medical problems, e.g. diabetes, heart disease, high blood pressure, epilepsy Obstetric and menstrual history in women	
Drug history	Current medications and effectiveness Immunisation status (in children or when clinically relevant)	
Social history	Smoking (or other tobacco use) – quantify in pack-years Alcohol consumption (type, amount, frequency, duration) and any symptoms of dependency Illicit drug use Exercise Housing and conditions Faith or spiritual history	
Family history	Red flags: tuberculosis, human immunodeficiency virus (HIV/AIDS), cancers, anaemia, diabetes, heart disease, myocardial infarction, hypertension, chronic obstructive pulmonary disease, asthma, stroke, renal disease, bleeding diseases, allergies, arthritis, alcohol abuse, mental illness	
Review of systems	See **Table 1.6**	

Table 1.1 History taking: a summary

You will soon learn key phrases to try to bring them back to the task in hand, e.g. 'Coming back to your chest pain, have you noticed …'.

Questions can be classified as either open or closed:

- **Open questions** (e.g. 'Why don't you tell me what's been going on?') are non-directive and allow the patient to give information freely. Patients can report information that is most important to them and also give their own version of events, in their own words. Open questions will work only if you are ready to take the time to listen. Use active listening (see below) to encourage the patient to keep speaking
- **A closed question** is one that elicits an answer such as 'yes', 'no' or something else factual, e.g. 'Does the pain move from your chest into your neck?'.

Use a funnelled approach to your consultation, starting with open questions and leading into closed questions.

Active listening

Active listening is a way to show patients that you are taking a genuine interest in what they are saying. This will not only make them feel valued, and improve the doctor–patient relationship, but

> ## Clinical insight
>
> All health professionals should be expert rapport builders. Good rapport is essential for patients being able to open their lives and their stories to you. Take your time to gain good rapport with patients.

will also encourage them to be honest and forthcoming. Here are a few key ways of listening actively:

- Lean forward
- Make eye contact
- Nod
- Repeat back what they have said, e.g. 'So you first noticed the problem 3 days ago?'
- Say 'mmm' or 'okay' to acknowledge what they have said

1.2 General principles of history taking

Over time you will develop your own style for taking a history. There are, however, key areas that must be covered, these include (**Table 1.1**):

- presenting complaint (PC)
- history of presenting complaint (HPC)
- past medical and surgical history (PMH/PSH)
- drug history (DH)
- family history (FH)
- social history (SH)
- ideas, concerns and effects or expectations (ICEs)
- review of systems

Taking a history is an inexact process. Two histories from the same patient on two different occasions will not necessarily be the same. For example, after a history has been taken, a patient may report new or completely different symptoms when a colleague joins the consultation.

Environment

The environment within which the consultation is undertaken is important. Most of your studies will take place in hospitals, but most consultations occur in outpatient or family medicine clinics. The environment should be comfortable and secure. On a ward, curtains offer little confidentiality and this should be taken into consideration when taking the patient's history, because he or she will be unlikely to disclose embarrassing or intimate information. Position yourself in an open and non-threatening position. Standing over a patient can be intimidating. Try not to position desks or beds between you and the patient. Use space in a way that makes the patient the centre of your attention. If consulting a threatening patient, never position the patient between yourself and the exit.

Clinical insight

HPC is sometimes known as the presenting problem (PB) and history of presenting problem (HPB). There is no one correct terminology and different teams will follow different trends.

Presenting complaint

The PC is the problem – or set of problems – that caused the patient to seek help from a doctor. Patients will often have more than one problem and each of these should be listed one by one. A good opening question might be 'What seems to be the problem today?'.

History of the presenting complaint

Take your time to elicit details on each of the presenting problems. As you take more histories you will become skilled at directing the consultation based on the information the patient gives you. Initially it may be worth memorising a useful mnemonic such as **OPERATES+** to ensure that key points are not missed (**Table 1.2**). Obtain details for each of the presenting problems. As you progress through the history, further problems may be identified that the patient did not initially report or identify as problematic. When a patient has several problems, it can be helpful to say that you will go through each problem in turn. That way each issue can be explored systematically and thoroughly without missing anything. A useful mnemonic for taking a pain history is **SOCRATES** (**Table 1.3**); this will identify all areas related to pain, but miss key features in alternative presentations.

	Mnemonic	Example questions
O	Onset of complaint	When did the problem start?
P	Progress of complaint	Has it always been the same?
E	Exacerbating factors	Is there anything that makes it worse?
R	Relieving factors	Is there anything that makes it better?
A	Associated symptoms	When you get this problem, do you notice any other symptoms?
T	Timing	Is there any time of day that you notice this problem more? How long does each episode last?
E	Episodes of recovery/ever before	Have you had this problem before? How often do you feel like this?
S	Severity	How bad is it?
+	Function	Does it prevent you from doing particular activities?

Table 1.2 OPERATES+: mnemonic for asking about presenting complaints

	Mnemonic	Example questions
S	Site	Where is the pain?
O	Onset	When did the pain start?
C	Character	Describe the pain to me, e.g. is it aching, shooting, stabbing or dull?
R	Radiation	Does the pain move to anywhere else in your body?
A	Associated symptoms	Have you had any symptoms other than the pain?
T	Timing	Pattern of pain (including time of day, frequency) Duration of pain Is it constant or does it come and go?
E	Exacerbating or relieving factors	Have you noticed anything that makes the pain better or worse?
S	Severity	Does the pain interfere with what you are doing? Does it keep you awake? If 0–10 is a scale of pain, with 0 as no pain and 10 as the worse pain that you can imagine, what score would you give this pain?

Table 1.3 SOCRATES: mnemonic for taking a pain history

Past medical history and past surgical history

Some clinicians prefer to take the PMH before the HPC. This enables them to develop a clear sense of what are current and what are past problems. If you choose to do so, explain to the patient: 'Before we discuss why you came today, I wanted to ask you some background questions. Would that be okay?'.

Start by asking an open question such as 'Have you had any serious illness in the past?'. Patients will often omit or forget important information. This is often because of the way in which a question is posed. Use several different questions to ensure that the patient understands. Similarly, use several different questions to elicit the past surgical history, e.g. 'Have you ever seen a surgeon?', 'Have you had any operations?' and/or 'Have you ever had an anaesthetic?'.

Specific past medical history

To finish, it is worthwhile asking a series of closed questions to identify any common or significant problems. A useful mnemonic is **JADE CAT MARCH (Table 1.4)**.

Drug history, allergies and immunisations

Drug history

It can be useful to start this section with the questions 'Do you have your medications with you' or 'Do you have a copy of your prescription?'. Patients often find it

> ## Clinical insight
>
> Do not be afraid of silence. Having asked an open question, give the patient time to respond. Allowing a pause after the patient has spoken may lead to him or her divulging more information. This is an invaluable time to employ active listening.

difficult to remember the medications they are taking or have taken in the past. Taking a drug history can therefore be one of the most difficult parts of the history.

It is essential to know:

- which medication(s) they are currently taking
- which medication(s) they have previously taken
- why each medication was started

General (JADE)	Respiratory (CAT)	Cardiovascular (MARCH)
J – jaundice	**C** – COPD	**M** – MI
A – anaemia	**A** – asthma	**A** – angina
D – diabetes	**T** – tuberculosis	**R** – rheumatic fever
E – epilepsy		**C** – CVA (stroke/TIA)
		H – hypertension
COPD, chronic obstructive pulmonary disease; CVA, cerebrovascular accident; TIA, transient ischaemia attack.		

Table 1.4 JADE CAT MARCH: mnemonic for important past medical history

- at what dose it/they have been prescribed
- in what preparation(s) it is given
- the effect that the medication(s) has had

In addition, identify:

- inhaler, cream, patch or suppository use
- any over-the-counter medications
- herbal and complementary medications
- any medications prescribed for somebody else but taken by the patient
- contraception – including implants and injections (patient's don't often think of these as medications)

Use this opportunity to check for compliance by asking patients if they take their medications as prescribed, e.g. 'How often do you forget to take your medicines?'. This is important for medications that may have been stopped by the patient because they have had 'no effect'. This can become evident for the first time in a patient who is admitted to a ward and has supervised medication administration, e.g. an elderly patient's blood pressure drops because the nurses start administering a high-dose β blocker that the patient has not been taking at home.

> ## Clinical insight
>
> Always clarify patients' understanding when they use medical jargon or diagnostic terms. They may mean something very different from the established medical meaning. 'Migraine' is a common example of this; patients often say that they have a migraine when really they mean a painful headache. Do not take these medical terms at face value; always explore what they mean when they use them.

Patients may be taking several different medications, each with its own side-effect profile. This can add to the symptoms that they have and also cloud your differential diagnosis.

Allergies

Reactions to drugs can range from life-threatening anaphylaxis through to mild side effects that have been misinterpreted by the patient. Ask the patient several questions to clarify this part of the history:

- 'Do you have any allergies?'
- 'Have you ever had a reaction to a medicine that you have taken?'

Immunisations

An immunisation history should be taken if it is relevant to the case. This is particularly important in children. For an elderly patient or anyone with chronic disease, ask if he or she has had the influenza (flu) immunisation. The World Health Organization recommends a minimum schedule of immunisations in all countries, with extended schedules for country-specific diseases.

Family history

Ask questions such as: 'Are there any illnesses that run in your family?' or 'Has anyone in your family had a similar problem?'. Taking a family history can also help identify any concerns that the patient may have.

How to draw a family tree

If necessary, draw a family tree (**Figure 1.1**) to help map the possible inheritance of the disease.

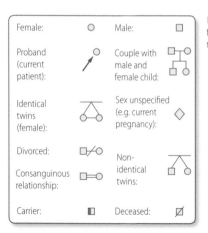

Figure 1.1 Symbols used for constructing a family tree.

Social history

Determine:

- employment (past and present)
- housing type and with whom the patient lives
- social support
- restrictive or unusual diets
- stresses at home and/or work
- restrictions on activities

You may wish to ask about the patient's faith, finances and hobbies if relevant. A good understanding of the patient's background will aid in forming a diagnosis and an appropriate management plan.

Clinical insight

A patient's lifestyle can have a significant impact on health. Many of the questions that you ask may be personal in nature but could have important implications for making an accurate diagnosis. Start by telling the patient 'I'm going to ask you some private questions which could be important'. Reassure the patient that what he or she reports will remain confidential to the medical team.

Ask about:

- foreign travel (it may be important to ask about sex tourism)
- alcohol and smoking history
- sexual history and/or sexual preferences
- illicit drug use (including type of drugs, method of use, volume of use)
- tattoos and body piercings

Basic activities of daily living and instrumental activities of daily living

Basic activities of daily living (BADLs) (**Table 1.5**) are used to describe a patient's functionality in self-care tasks. Instrumental activities of daily living (IADLs) describe the ability to maintain an independent household. If a patient is unable to perform any of these tasks, it is important to identify what factors are limiting the ability to do so. These assessments are not only good measures of how a disease is impacting on a patient, but also of the support he or she will need in order to return home independently.

Faith or spiritual history

Taking a faith history requires permission, sensitivity and respect. Not only does it help us to know more about our patients, but it also

Basic activities of daily living	Instrumental activities of daily living
Bathing, personal hygiene and grooming Dressing and undressing Toileting Transferring and mobility Continence Feeding	Shopping for groceries Driving or using public transportation Using a telephone Undertaking housework Completing home repair Preparing meals Laundry Taking medications Handling finances

Table 1.5 Activities of daily living

guides decision-making during the practice of evidence-based medicine (e.g. a Muslim may wish to be offered low-molecular-weight heparin that is non-porcine in origin).

How to take a faith or spiritual history Here are some examples of appropriate questions to ask patients about their spiritual 'health':

1. 'It would help me to treat you better if I knew more about you.'
2. 'Do you have a personal faith that helps you (in a time like this)? How does it affect your life?'
3. 'Do you belong to a faith community? Some people find it helpful to meet with someone. Would you like us to arrange this for you?'

Smoking, alcohol and illicit substance use
Smoking – what is a pack-year?

Quantify smoking in terms of pack-years: 20 cigarettes per day for 1 year equates to 1 pack-year (e.g. 15 cigarettes per day for 4 years is equivalent to 3 pack-years). Also ask about other tobacco products.

Clinical insight

Ask: 'Do you or have you ever smoked?' Many smokers will say that they are non-smokers if they stopped recently.

Alcohol

The effects of alcohol on health are enormous, including acute intoxication and chronic disease (e.g. liver disease and psychiatric problems such as addiction and depression). Alcohol also leads to social problems such as reduced productivity, violent crimes and antisocial behaviour. Many patients who are alcohol dependent will enter a stage of withdrawal in hospital if this area is not appropriately investigated. Ask questions such as:

1. 'How much do you drink each week?'
2. 'Have you ever been a heavy drinker?'
3. 'What is the most that you will drink in one go?'

When documenting the history, report alcohol use in units per week and state if evidence of bingeing is present. One unit of alcohol is equivalent to 10 mL of pure alcohol, so:

$$\text{Units of alcohol} = \text{Alcohol by volume (\%)} \times \text{Volume of alcohol (mL)} \div 1000.$$

Therefore 125 mL glass of 14% white wine is equivalent to 1.75 units alcohol. Be sure to clarify how much a patient means; for example when a patient says 'a whisky a night' is this a standard 25 mL measure or a larger shot poured by the patient? A simple and non-judgmental way of asking this is 'How quickly do you finish a 75 cL sized bottle of whisky?'.

CAGE questionnaire This is a quick and easy method for assessing possible alcohol dependence. Two 'yes' responses indicate that the possibility of alcoholism should be investigated further:

- **C** – Have you ever felt that you needed to cut down on your drinking?
- **A** – Have people annoyed you by criticising your drinking?
- **G** – Have you ever felt guilty about drinking?
- **E** – Have you ever felt that you needed a drink first thing in the morning (eye-opener) to steady your nerves or to get rid of a hangover?

Binge drinking (heavy episodic drinking) is drinking heavily in a short space of time in order to get drunk or feel the effects of alcohol. It can be loosely defined as twice the daily recommended limit, i.e. 8 units in men, 6 units in women.

Illicit drugs

Reassure patients that any information they give you is confidential. Asking direct questions will often lead to an immediate denial, so indirect questioning can be useful e.g. 'What drugs have your friends tried?', '... and you?'. Once you have gained the patient's confidence, establish:

- which illicit drugs have been used
- when and for how long
- how much and how often
- how they were taken (i.e. orally, smoked, injected venously, injected subcutaneously)
- what the impact has been on his or her health and life

Clinical insight

There are only rare times when doctors can and should break patient confidentiality:

- disclosures required by law (e.g. certain infectious diseases)
- disclosures required in the public interest
- to protect the patient (if not practicable to seek a patient's consent)
- to protect others (if failure to do so may expose others to a risk of death or serious harm).

Always inform the patient that you are informing someone of his or her condition unless doing so could cause harm (e.g. safeguarding children).

Nutrition

There is a clear association between nutrition and health. A nutrition history may be necessary if a patient is undernourished or overweight. A good nutrition history is important for giving lifestyle advice as part of preventive medicine.

Nutrition history

1. How many meals and snacks do you eat each day?
2. How many times a week do you eat away from home? What do you eat?
3. On average, how many pieces of fruit or glasses of juice do you eat or drink each day?
4. On average, how many servings of vegetables do you eat each day?
5. How much fibre do you eat?
6. How many times a week do you eat red meat, chicken and/or fish?

7. How many hours of television do you watch each day? Do you snack during viewing?
8. How many times a week do you eat desserts and/or sweets?
9. What types of beverages do you drink, how much and how often?
10. How much alcohol do you drink?

Review of systems

Start with a statement such as: 'I am now going to ask you some specific questions'. A comprehensive list of symptoms is given in **Table 1.6**. It would be almost impossible to go through the entire list with all patients. As you start learning to take histories try to be as comprehensive as possible. With time your ability to focus your review of systems, dependent upon the HPC, will improve. Use lay terms when questioning the patient.

Ideas, concerns and effects or expectations

Explore the patient's ICEs. Although this is part of the history, some clinicians ask about ICEs at the end of the consultation, once they have examined the patient and before discussing the management. This is a matter of discretion.

Ideas
- 'Have you got any thoughts about what could be causing your symptoms?'

Concerns
- 'Is there anything in particular that you had in mind when you came to the clinic today?'
- 'Is there anything in particular that is worrying you about your symptoms?'

Effects or expectations
- 'Was there anything that you were hoping we might be able to do for you today?'
- 'Did you have any particular tests or treatments in mind that you were expecting us to organise?'

General	generally well or unwell weight loss or gain appetite loss or gain fevers, sweats or rigors level of activity	fatigue change in mood rashes or bruising 'lumps or bumps'
Respiratory	cough shortness of breath wheeze	sputum haemoptysis frequent chest infections
Genitourinary	urinary symptoms: dysuria, frequency, urgency, nocturia ease of passage of urine haematuria	urethral discharge sexual function menstrual cycle
Cardiovascular	chest pain shortness of breath orthopnoea nocturnal dyspnoea oedema	palpitations claudication collapse exercise tolerance
Nervous system	headaches fits, faints or funny turns weakness (or unsteadiness) dizziness or loss of balance changes or loss in vision, hearing or taste	transient loss of function (e.g. vision, speech or sight) paraesthesiae muscle wasting involuntary movements urinary incontinence
Gastrointestinal	nausea and vomiting haematemesis dyspepsia dysphagia odynophagia	abdominal pain, mass or swelling bowel pattern diarrhoea or constipation rectal bleeding jaundice or itchy skin
Musculoskeletal	weakness change in mobility stiffness	joint pain or swelling or erythema

Table 1.6 Systems review (adult patients)

Common pitfalls in history taking

There are many pitfalls that can reduce your chances of obtaining an accurate history. Groopman describes three common pitfalls

Clinical insight

Doctors are often fearful to ask the question: 'Can you think of anything to explain what is going on?', worrying that this is a sign of our diagnostic weakness. Patients often have a very good explanation for their symptoms. However, at times, their perception can be very poor and this is an opportunity to address their ideas, concerns and effects.

Clinical insight

Common pitfalls in history taking include:

- Using medical terminology or complex language
- Asking leading questions or 'framing' questions to obtain a desired response (e.g. 'Is the pain sharp' rather than 'What does the pain feel like?')
- Using too many closed questions
- Stacking questions (i.e. too many questions together)
- Failing to clarify information
- Interrupting patients or not giving undivided attention
- Casting immediate judgements on the patient that affect your interpretation of the information given
- Failing to summarise the history back to the patient
- More attention given to note taking than listening to the patient

made by clinicians when taking a history.

1. Anchoring

This occurs when doctors latch onto an early piece of information, e.g. if the nurse says 'Can you see the patient with asthma in room 4', they then focus their history around this early suspicion of asthma. They ask closed questions that confirm their early suspicion of asthma and minimise other symptoms or signs that may suggest that the diagnosis is something different.

2. Availability

You may have recently seen a case that is particularly dramatic, or lots of cases of a particular diagnosis, so may fall into the pitfall of availability, e.g. having recently seen several cases of oesophagitis, you may falsely diagnose your next patient with chest pain as having oesophagitis.

3. Attribution

You may immediately make judgements about a patient on first encounter, e.g. if a 22-year-old student presents with vaginal discharge, you may falsely assume that she has a sexually transmitted infection.

Clinical examination

Examination of the patient is covered in Chapters 2–14. Before progressing to the examination, it is worthwhile summarising the history back to the patient. This will give him or her the opportunity to confirm whether your version of events is correct and will provide reassurance that you have listened to all of the problems.

1.3 Forming a differential diagnosis

The differential diagnosis

The aim of the history and examination is to formulate a diagnosis while also planning possible investigations and treatments. A differential diagnosis is a systematic approach used to identify the true diagnosis among many other alternatives, known as the 'differential diagnoses' or 'differentials'.

There are a series of steps in formulating and acting on a list of differential diagnoses:

1. Gather all the information from the history and examination to form a list (mental or written) of symptoms and signs
2. List all the possible causes for these symptoms and signs
3. Prioritise this list based on the most urgent or life threatening and those that are statistically the most likely
4. List investigations and treatments that should be drawn up, which will either confirm or rule out diagnoses, while treating any active or life-threatening symptoms

This is a complex process of mental reasoning and will take skilled clinicians years to perfect. Using a mnemonic ('surgical sieve') can be useful in helping to draw up a list of differential diagnoses.

An easy mnemonic for remembering a surgical sieve is **VITAMIN CDE**:

V – vascular, **I** – inflammatory (infectious and non-infectious), **T** – trauma/toxins, **A** – autoimmune, **M** – metabolic, **I** – idiopathic, **N** – neoplastic, **C** -congenital, **D** – degenerative, **E** – environmental.

Multiple causation

Symptoms and signs will rarely give a single clear diagnosis that immediately responds to a single treatment. Often symptoms can be multi-factorial in nature, e.g. a patient may have lower back pain due to a strained muscle and depression. The depression causes an exacerbation of the symptoms of the back pain, in turn exacerbating the depression because the patient may stop leaving home because of the pain.

Clinical insight

Globally, there are a number of diseases that continue to claim a large proportion of lives each year.

Adults	Children
Ischaemic heart disease	Pneumonia
Stroke and other cerebrovascular disease	Prematurity
Lower respiratory infections	Diarrhoeal diseases
Chronic obstructive pulmonary disease	Birth complications (asphyxia)
Diarrhoeal diseases	Malaria
HIV/AIDS	Undernutrition
Trachea, bronchus, lung cancers	Injuries
Tuberculosis	HIV/AIDS
Diabetes mellitus	Measles
Road traffic accidents	Congenital diseases

Management

The term 'management' is used to describe a combination of the investigations and treatments that are offered to the patient. Document which investigations you would like to perform and what treatments you would like to start immediately.

Planning investigations

Investigations are tests that can be used to define and measure the extent of a diagnosis and/or measure the progress of a disease and the response to treatment. Investigations should be ordered carefully based on the differentials. Patients should not receive a 'blanket' series of tests in the hope of unearthing something. Rather the investigations ordered should be rationalised and justified. When deciding which investigations to order, one should consider the following:

- How will the results affect the management of the patient?
- Are there any risks to the test?
- What specimens will need to be taken and is it possible in this patient?
- Does the cost of the test warrant its use?
- How quickly should the test be arranged?

1.4 After the consultation

At the end of any consultation explain to the patient:
- what you have found during the history and examination
- what the likely diagnosis is and any possible alternatives (differentials)
- what tests, if any, are required, what they involve and how accurate they are
- what treatments can be started, how these work, how they are taken and what side effects may be seen

Documenting in medical notes

It is very important to write good notes that are contemporaneous (**Figure 1.2**). In doing so it will help process your thoughts and plans, record what has been done and aid communication with your colleagues.

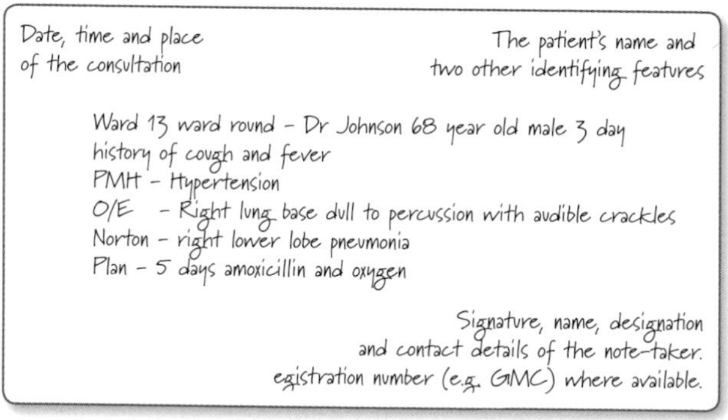

Date, time and place of the consultation

The patient's name and two other identifying features

Ward 13 ward round – Dr Johnson 68 year old male 3 day history of cough and fever
PMHt – Hypertension
O/E – Right lung base dull to percussion with audible crackles
Norton – right lower lobe pneumonia
Plan – 5 days amoxicillin and oxygen

Signature, name, designation and contact details of the note-taker. egistration number (e.g. GMC) where available.

Figure 1.2 Contemporaneous notes.

During the first consultation, often referred to as 'the clerking', the documentation will follow the same structure as the consultation, i.e. PC, HPC PMH, DH, FH, SH, examination, differentials, management. Documentation is said to be contemporaneous if it is made at the time of, or as soon as possible after, the consultation (**Figure 1.2**).

Presenting patients to colleagues

Once you have mastered the skills of taking a history and examining a patient, you will need to learn and practise how to present this information to your colleagues and seniors. This is important for your own learning but also for improving patient care. Presenting a case should follow the same structure as the consultation (**Figure 1.3**).

1.5 Evidence-based medicine

What is evidence-based medicine and why is it relevant to clinical skills?

Evidence-based medicine (EBM) is the integration of the current best research evidence (e.g. journal articles) with our own clinical expertise, along with the values that are unique to our patients. A common misconception is that EBM is a process of substituting our clinical expertise with research. In reality EBM is a process that combines three key principles:

1. Clinical expertise
2. Patient values, circumstances, expectations and beliefs
3. Best available research evidence

Key principles of EBM

Clinical expertise

Clinical skills are enhanced by the experience of seeing patients. Underpinned by good communication skills, a thorough history and examination not only assist with differential diagnosis but also allow you to ascertain the patient's personal values and expectations. It is impossible to practise EBM without good clinical skills, e.g. without a correct clinical diagnosis, a clinician will search the wrong research evidence.

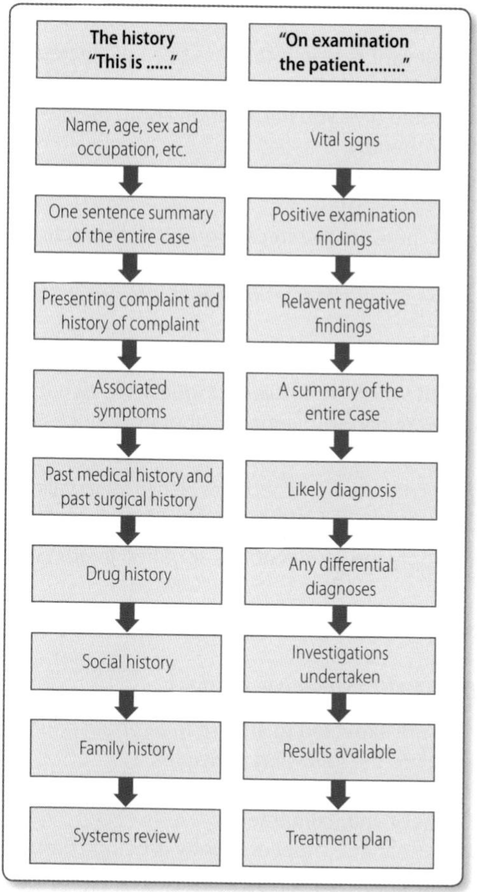
The history
"This is ......"
Name, age, sex and occupation, etc.
One sentence summary of the entire case
Presenting complaint and history of complaint
Associated symptoms
Past medical history and past surgical history
Drug history
Social history
Family history
Systems review
"On examination the patient........."
Vital signs
Positive examination findings
Relavent negative findings
A summary of the entire case
Likely diagnosis
Any differential diagnoses
Investigations undertaken
Results available
Treatment plan

Figure 1.3 Presenting to colleagues and seniors.

Patient values, circumstances, expectations and beliefs

Patient values are the unique preferences, concerns and expectations that each patient brings to each clinical encounter. These must be woven into clinical decisions to best serve the patient, e.g. the patient with hypertension in **Figure 1.4** may have osteoarthritis and find an exercise ECG painful and stressful.

Best research evidence

This is clinically relevant research that has been evaluated to assess whether it is of high quality and that it is directly relevant to the patient. It could give you information about diagnostic tests, prognosis or therapy.

Five steps for practising EBM

Sackett states that there are five steps (**Figure 1.4**) in practising EBM:

Step 1 – Ask: convert our information needs into answerable questions

Step 2 – Acquire: track down, with maximum efficiency, the best evidence with which to answer our questions (whether from the clinical examination, diagnostic laboratory, published literature or other sources)

Step 3 – Appraise: critically appraise this evidence for its validity (closeness to the truth) and usefulness (clinical applicability)

Step 4 – Apply: apply the results of this appraisal in our clinical practice

Step 5 – Assess: evaluate our performance

1.6 Ethicolegal considerations

As a clinician you are expected to adhere to a certain code of practice. This involves the following principles:

- Keep your knowledge and skills up to date, always working within the limits of your competence
- If you think that patient safety or dignity is being compromised, take prompt action
- Always treat patients as individuals and maintain confidentiality
- Work in partnership with the patients, enabling them to make decisions about their care
- Finally, never discriminate unfairly against patients or colleagues, or abuse a patient's trust.

Clinical problem:
A 68-year-old man who is overweight and hypertensive presents with a history of recurrent episodes of chest pain and shortness of breath. You would like to know if a standard ECG is likely to miss any pathology.

Step 1: Ask a PICO question	**Patient, population or problem** Adult with hypertension	**Intervention** Standard/rest electrocardiogram (ECG)	**Control** Stress/ exercise ECG	**Outcome** Correct diagnosis of angina

Step 2: Acquire relevant information	Use online resources, books and review papers

Step 3: Appraise the evidence	• Relevance • Validity • Significance • Applicability

Step 4: Apply the results to your patient	Use the evidence you have found to investigate or treat the patient. Applying the results is dependent upon the judgements made in the appraisal of the evidence

Step 5: Evaluate your performance	As clinicians we should always be asking the question: 'Am I doing the best thing for my patient?' This could involve personal reflection or systematic processes such as audit or quality.

Figure 1.4 Evidence-based medicine.

In the UK this is outlined by the General Medical Council's *Duties of a Doctor*.

Four pillars of medical ethics

There are four pillars of medical ethics: autonomy, beneficence, non-maleficence and justice. Doctors should also reflect on the scope of application of these principles.

Autonomy

Autonomy is the capacity for self-determination. It is the right to choose what you want, for yourself, in an unbiased environment. A decision made by an individual may not appear rational but this does not mean that the individual is therefore incapable of acting autonomously or that he or she does not have capacity.

Beneficence

Beneficence is the concept of acting to benefit an individual or a population. In treating a patient autonomously consider that one patient's beneficence may be another patient's maleficence.

Non-maleficence

Non-maleficence is the concept of 'doing no harm', e.g. stopping a medication that has no benefit but has side effects. Whenever doctors try to benefit a patient (beneficence) there is always the possibility that they may harm them (maleficence); there should always be a 'net benefit' for the patient.

Justice

Practise in a manner that is fair to all. This should include distributive justice (the fair distribution of resources), respect for people's rights and respect for morally acceptable laws.

Other ethical principles

Best interests

Work with colleagues in ways that best serve patients' interests.

Confidentiality

All parts of the medical consultation are confidential. There are few cases when confidentiality can be relaxed (page 13).

Capacity

In order to have capacity, a patient must be able to:
- understand the information relevant to the decision
- retain the information
- use that information as part of the decision-making process
- communicate his or her decision by talking or signing, or by any other means

Key legal concepts

Legal standards vary in different countries. The concepts here describe the general principles that are held to be true in the UK.

Consent

Consent is the process of gaining approval or permission after thoughtful consideration. Consent can be implied, verbal or written. Consent is valid if: (1) the patient has capacity, (2) the patient was sufficiently informed, and (3) the consent was voluntary and not coerced. Consent is often regarded as a legal expression of autonomy.

Decisions relating to cardiopulmonary resuscitation

Respect the desires of well-informed patients who do not wish to undergo cardiopulmonary resuscitation. This may appear to be a difficult consultation, but most patients who are near the end of life will have a desire to discuss the pertinent issues. It will also often open a door to a discussion between a patient and their loved ones about their current clinical condition. Clinicians should assist their patients in this discussion.

Personal beliefs

In order to treat a patient autonomously, you must treat patients with respect whatever their life choices and beliefs. You must not unfairly discriminate against them by allowing your personal views to adversely affect your professional relationship with them or the treatment that you provide or arrange.

Probity

Probity means being honest and trustworthy and acting with integrity; this is at the heart of medical professionalism.

General principles of examination

The examination should be focused, based on the findings from the patient's history. Examining a patient is a scientific skill and yet it is also an art form. It is used to elicit important clinical findings but also as physical contact between a vulnerable patient and a physician. Most clinical examinations follow a very regimented structure, which is covered in this chapter.

2.1 General structure of examination

Examination should always follow a clear structure. Start by preparing yourself as follows:

- Ensure that all the required equipment is available
- Wash your hands
- Ensure that there is privacy
- Introduce yourself to the patient and gain verbal consent for the examination
- Ensure that there is a clean sheet on the bed and position the patient comfortably
- Expose the necessary areas to be examined, at the appropriate times, while maintaining patient dignity to the best of your ability

Here is a general structure for the subsequent examination:

- note vital signs
- general inspection
- palpation
- percussion
- any relevant auscultation
- complete the examination with any final assessments, e.g. an ear, nose and throat (ENT) examination
- thank the patient and cover and/or help him or her to dress

2.2 Preparation for the examination

Wash hands

The first principle is do no harm. Good hand hygiene prevents the spread of infectious conditions. Wash your hands immediately before and after examining a patient. Hands should be washed with alcohol rub, or soap and water if they are dirty, or if the patient has gastroenteritis.

Introduce yourself to the patient and gain consent for the examination

Introduce yourself, giving your name and designation. Explain to the patient what the examination will involve and ask for his or her consent to proceed. The consent for an examination is usually implied (Chapter 1), e.g. 'Hello, my name is John Smith. I am a first year medical student. My senior has asked me to come in and examine your abdomen. Is that alright with you?'.

Ensure privacy

Always ensure that the patient is given the dignity of having the examination performed in private. Bear in mind that hospital curtains do not offer much confidentiality. Wherever possible, offer the patient the security of having an impartial observer (a chaperone) present during an intimate examination. This applies whether or not you are the same gender as the patient.

Position the patient

The position of the patient depends on the system being examined:
- 45° for cardiovascular
- 90° for respiratory
- supine for abdominal

It may be difficult to attain the correct position in critically ill or elderly patients and, in this case, carry out the examination to the best of your ability in a position that is safe and comfortable for the patient, accounting for the limitations in your findings.

Examine the patient from the patient's right side

It is traditional to examine from the patient's right-hand side. This is to allow your dominant right hand to palpate effectively. If you are left-handed, then examine from the patient's left side. Be sure to explain this to an examiner who might otherwise think that you are inexperienced at examining patients. The choice of side may also be dictated by the position of the couch against any walls.

Expose the area being examined

Once the peripheries have been examined, it will be necessary to further expose the patient. Never examine the patient through clothing because this often leads to erroneous or missed findings. Allow the patient to undress in private and provide a gown or sheet. During the examination, maintain the patient's dignity by covering any body parts that are not being directly examined. Classically, for abdominal examination, it has been said that the patient should be exposed 'from nipple to knees'. However, this can be embarrassing for the patient; the genitalia should be examined independently once the abdomen has been examined.

> ### Clinical insight
>
> There are different approaches used for performing any one examination. There is often no 'right' or 'wrong' way. Moreover, it is vital that you use a system that is consistent and well practised. In this book we have set a pattern that we feel is comprehensive and easy to reproduce.

> ### Clinical insight
>
> As a clinician, vital signs (or 'observations') will normally have been performed by nursing or clinical support staff. However, it is important that you know how to carry out these simple, yet crucial, measurements yourself.

2.3 Vital signs (observations)

Vital signs can be taken either at the start or at the end of the examination. Ensure that the patient is comfortable and at rest when you assess these. The vital signs can also be used to assess the global wellbeing of the patient using an early warning score (EWS) (**Figure 15.1**).

Trends of vital signs are of more use than an individual assessment, e.g. a blood pressure (BP) of 87/50 mmHg is concerning, although, if over the past 5 days the BP measurements were 90/55 mmHg, you would be far less concerned.

Pulse rate, rhythm, volume and character

Use your index and middle fingers to feel the radial pulse (Chapter 3). Assess it for the following:

- Rate: count the pulse for 15 seconds, then multiply this by 4 in order to calculate the number of **beats per minute** (beats/min or bpm)
- Rhythm: the rhythm should be regular; the pulse rate can increase with inspiration, which can give the impression of irregularity (sinus arrhythmia)
- Character and volume: assess at the carotid artery
- Delay: radioradial and radiofemoral

Respiratory rate

This is a very important clinical sign that is often neglected. Count the respiratory rate over 1 minute to get an accurate number of **respirations per minute**. It is helpful to pretend to continue to take the radial pulse while doing this (if patients think that you are monitoring their breathing then they will often subconsciously change their rate or pattern). While counting the respiratory rate, simultaneously assess the work of breathing – it should be regular.

Abnormal patterns of respiration

These can give important indicators of the general clinical condition of the patient while also leading to a potential diagnosis. **Cheyne–Stokes respiration** (also known as periodic respiration) is a cycle of deep and shallow respiration with occasional apnoeas. This is a poor prognostic sign often seen in terminal care. **Paroxysmal nocturnal dyspnoea** is acute dyspnoea, causing the patient to wake from sleep; sitting upright or standing will lead to relief. This is associated with pulmonary oedema caused by left ventricular failure. **Kussmaul's respiration** is deep sighing respiration associated with metabolic acidosis, e.g. diabetic ketoacidosis. **Air hunger** is acute dyspnoea found in the terminal stages of an exsanguinating haemorrhage. It is a serious sign, indicating that immediate intervention is needed. **Obstructive sleep apnoea** is due to intermittent and repeated periods of upper airway collapse during sleep, causing apnoea, often associated with obesity. Patients often present with daytime sleepiness due to poor sleep at night.

Temperature

Assess for a significant pyrexia (>38.5°C) or hypothermia (<35°C).

Fever

This is an elevation in core body temperature (**Table 2.1**). It is a presenting feature in most infections but is also found in autoimmune and inflammatory conditions. Temperature

Cardiovascular	Infective endocarditis, thromboembolic, e.g. pulmonary embolism
Respiratory	Upper or lower respiratory tract infection, tuberculosis, empyema
Gastrointestinal tract and pelvis	Abdominal or pelvic abscess, urinary tract infections, pelvic inflammatory disease, inflammatory bowel disease, pancreatitis
Neurological	Meningitis (bacterial or viral), encephalitis, brain damage (disordered thermoregulation), brain haemorrhage
Musculoskeletal	Osteomyelitis, septic arthritis, juvenile idiopathic arthritis
Connective tissue disorders	Rheumatoid arthritis, systemic lupus erythematosus, giant cell arteritis, polyarteritis nodosa
Malignancies	Lung cancer, leukaemia, lymphoma, renal cell carcinoma
Other	Other infections: septicaemia, viral (e.g. HIV), bacterial (e.g. acute otitis media), protozoal (e.g. malaria) Drugs (e.g. antimicrobials), dental abscess, hyperthyroidism, phaeochromocytoma, tissue destruction, (e.g. surgery), infarction, allergic conditions, transfusion reactions

Table 2.1 Common and/or important causes of fever

is controlled by the thermoregulatory centre in the anterior hypothalamus. During fever the 'thermostat setting' in the hypothalamus shifts upwards. **Hyperpyrexia** is the term used for a fever ≥41.5°C. This can occur in patients with severe infections but most commonly occurs in central nervous system (CNS) haemorrhages. **Rigor** is an extreme reflex response characterised by an episode of shaking or exaggerated shivering. Ask the patient specifically if he or she has had these symptoms because they can be suggestive of severe bacterial infection. **Pyrogens** are substances that cause fever; they may be **exogenous** (e.g. endotoxin from bacteria) or **endogenous** (e.g. cytokines). Pyrexia of unknown origin (PUO) is a fever of >38.3°C on several occasions for at least 3 weeks, of uncertain diagnosis after 1 week of investigation. This is a challenging assessment. If fever is found, then it should be classified as follows:

- **Continuous**: does not fluctuate >1°C in 24 hours
- **Intermittent**: present only for a certain period, later cycling back to normal
- **Remittent**: remains above normal throughout the day and fluctuates >1°C in 24 hours

Hypothermia
This is a low temperature that may be caused by:
- environmental exposure (e.g. near drowning or perioperative)
- secondary to a medical cause (e.g. hypothyroidism, sepsis or post-stroke)

Blood pressure
BP measurement is usually achieved using an automated (oscillometry) system. In hospitals these systems are usually connected to a monitor, although domiciliary devices with a built-in display are also available.

To measure BP manually, use a sphygmomanometer and follow this sequence:
1. Sit or lay the patient comfortably
2. Place the arm and sphygmomanometer at the same level as the heart

3. Ensure a correct inflatable cuff size: length 80% of upper arm encircling (width), >40% of the circumference; a short cuff will overestimate the BP and a long cuff will underestimate it

4. Place the centre of the inflatable bladder over the brachial artery and firmly secure the cuff

5. Locate the brachial pulse

> ## Clinical insight
>
> Korotkoff's sounds are heard as the sphygmomanometer cuff is deflated
>
> **Phase 1:** first appearance of the sounds (**systolic BP**)
>
> **Phases 2 and 3:** increasingly loud sounds
>
> **Phase 4:** abrupt muffling of the sounds
>
> **Phase 5:** disappearance of the sounds (**diastolic BP**)

6. Inflate the cuff to approximately 30 mmHg above the point when the brachial pulse disappeared

7. Place a stethoscope over the brachial artery and slowly reduce the pressure. Systolic pressure is noted when **Korotkoff's sounds** are first heard, and diastolic pressure is noted when the sounds disappear

If there is concern about **postural (orthostatic) hypotension**, ask the patient to stand for ≥1min before repeating the BP measurement. A systolic drop (on standing) of ≥20 mmHg or a diastolic drop of ≥10 mmHg indicates postural hypotension. If the BP is high, consider requesting **ambulatory blood pressure** (ABP) monitoring. This is a test that repeatedly measures BP with the patient at home over 24 hours.

Hypertension

This is high blood pressure. It is defined (on one-off BP) as:

- **pre-hypertension:** >120/80 mmHg
- **stage 1 hypertension:** ≥140/90 mmHg
- **stage 2 hypertension:** ≥160/100 mmHg
- **severe hypertension:** ≥180/110 mmHg

Capillary refill time

This is defined as the time taken to restore perfusion to the skin after a period of pressure. Using a finger or thumb, press on the sternum for 5 seconds and note the time for colour to return (blanch time) once the pressure has been released. A capillary nail refill time can be performed with the same method at the nail bed. The finger should be held at the same vertical position as the heart. A normal refill time is ≤2 s. A blanch time greater than this can indicate: dehydration, shock, hypothermia and/ or peripheral vascular disease. This test is more commonly performed in children but can also be useful in adults.

Pulse oximetry

Pulse oximetry (also known as oxygen saturation) is simple to perform, cheap and non-invasive. The pulse oximeter probes consist of two light-emitting diodes and a photodetector. These measure the percentage of haemoglobin that is 'bound to oxygen'. The probes are most commonly placed on fingers or earlobes. A normal oxygen saturation is 94–98% (**Table 2.2**), although levels of 88–92% are considered normal in people with chronic obstructive pulmonary disease (COPD). Pulse oximetry does not provide information about the true oxygen content of the blood, which is called the partial pressure of oxygen (Chapter 4). The relationship between oxygen saturation and the partial pressure of oxygen is not linear, so it is a useful but not completely accurate bedside test. The oxygen saturation can be inaccurate in hypothermia, poor perfusion, anaemia, carbon monoxide poisoning, excessive movement, or if nail varnish is present. Below 70%, oxygen saturation levels are not accurate.

Clinical insight

Frank cyanosis does not develop until the level of deoxyhaemoglobin reaches 5 g/dL, which corresponds to an arterial oxygen saturation (Sa_2O) of around 67%

Pulse rate	51–90 beats/min or bpm
Respiratory rate	12–20/min
Blood pressure – systolic	100–140 mmHg
Temperature (define if oral, etc.)	36.1–38.0°C
Blood oxygen saturation	94–98%

Table 2.2 Normal vital signs in adults

2.4 Techniques for examination

Inspection

Your examination begins as soon as you meet the patient. For general inspection always start at the foot of the bed and make observations about the patient and the setting. Make the patient comfortable on the couch or the bed. Inspect from head to toes and front to back; this will require adequate exposure of the patient.

Palpation

Palpation is used to locate anatomical landmarks, discern the range of movements of limbs, ascertain the texture of tissues and organs, assess masses and/or to investigate superficial or deep pain.

> **Clinical insight**
>
> There are variations of acceptability of touch in different cultural contexts. The arm is the most acceptable place to touch a patient. If you feel awkward or do not feel empathy, then you should not touch the patient except for examination purposes.

Touching a patient before gaining consent (normally implied or verbal) is an assault of that person. While gaining consent, always ask if the patient has pain. If there is a location that is painful, palpate that region last. Always watch the patient's face when palpating because this may reveal signs of pain that the patient doesn't report verbally.

Percussion

Percussion provides subjective information about the underlying structure. It can be direct or indirect. Direct percussion is performed by directly striking the patient (e.g. the clavicle) with your middle finger. Indirect percussion (also known as digitodigital percussion) is performed by placing your hand on the patient and then striking your own finger. Either will result in the production of one of several percussion notes:

- **resonant:** normal
- **hyperresonant (tympanic):** heard over areas of decreased density
- **dull:** heard over areas of increased density
- **stony dull:** extreme dullness (characteristic of pleural effusion)

To percuss indirectly (**Figure 2.1**) you need to do the following:
1. Relax all but the middle finger on the structure being percussed (e.g. chest wall)
2. Ensure that the middle finger is firmly placed to enable good sound transmission
3. Percuss the distal interphalangeal joint using your free hand (the movement comes from the wrist and not the elbow)
4. Percuss two to three times in short succession

Auscultation

Auscultation is the term used to describe the process of listening to the sounds made by internal organs. The heart, lungs and abdomen are most commonly auscultated, although the head of newborns (via the anterior fontanelle) and vascular swellings may also be auscultated. Auscultation involves using an instrument, mostly a stethoscope.

Clinical insight

The earpieces of the stethoscope should be placed facing forward to improve sound quality. This is because the ear canal runs posterior to anterior.

How to use a stethoscope

The stethoscope has a diaphragm and a bell. The diaphragm picks up high-frequency sounds and the bell low-frequency sounds (do not press too hard with the bell because it can become a diaphragm if used in this way). The diaphragm is mainly used because it gives greater

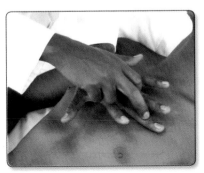

Figure 2.1 Chest percussion.

sound amplification. The bell is used in examining the neck and supraclavicular regions and for specific heart sounds.

2.5 General inspection

Make a note of any key signs on general examination (**Table 2.3**).

Inspection of the environment

Look around the patient's environment and bedside. Look for devices such as catheters, inhalers, sputum pots or medications. Is there oxygen being delivered? If so, how much and via what type of delivery device? (page 94)

General	Abnormal colour Looks unwell or in pain	Poor nutrition or hydration Abnormal breathing pattern
Environment	Medications, e.g. inhalers Intravenous drip Oxygen masks	Sputum pot Catheter
Vital signs	Hypo- or hypertension Tachy- or bradycardia Tachypnoea	Respiratory depression Hyper- or hypothermia Low oxygen saturation
Eyes	Jaundice Pallor	Unequal or unreactive pupils
Face	Characteristic facies	Asymmetry
Mouth	Poor dental hygiene Buccal lesions	Mouth odour Fungal infection
Neck	Lymphadenopathy Raised jugular venous pressure	Distended vessels Deviated trachea Goitre
Hands	Palmar colour Temperature Nail signs (including clubbing)	Deformity Tremor
Legs and feet	Oedema Colour change Peripheral pulses Dermatological	Skin lesions Abnormal colour Abnormal hair loss or growth

Table 2.3 Key signs on general examination

General appearance, comfort and breathing pattern

Ask the following questions to establish how sick the patient appears:

- Does the patient look well, unwell or very unwell? If they look very unwell the examination may need to be more focused (Chapter 15)
- Is the breathing rate and pattern normal? Assess symmetry by asking the patient to take one deep breath
- Is the patient using accessory muscles of respiration? Is the patient pale or cyanosed?
- Is the patient comfortable or distressed?

Colour

Is **pallor** (paleness), **cyanosis** (blueness) or **jaundice** (yellowness) present? Cyanosis can be central (the tongue appears blue) or peripheral (bluish discoloration elsewhere, e.g. fingers or around lips). Other abnormal colours include slate-grey appearance (seen in haemochromatosis) and darkened skinfolds and mucosa (seen in Addison's disease).

Mental and emotional state

Although a full mental and emotional state may need to be assessed as part of a psychiatric assessment (Chapter 11), it is possible to quickly gauge the patient's general mental and emotional state at the start of the consultation. This is important because it will guide how you approach the patient.

Nutrition

A good nutrition history is important (page 13). Clinically assess the patient's nutritional state. Does the patient look overweight, adequately nourished or malnourished? Weight can be classified according to the body mass index (BMI), which is measured as weight/height^2 (kg/m^2). The normal range is 18.5–24.9. BMI is not reliable in children as it is age and gender dependent. Rather, they should have their weight and height plotted on an age- and sex-appropriate growth chart. Arm-span is the measurement with the closest correlation to height and is useful in patients who can't have their height measured (e.g. bed bound).

Classification of BMI
- **<18.5**: underweight
- **18.5–24.9**: normal
- **25–29.9**: overweight
- **30–34.9**: class I obesity (severe obesity)
- **35–39.9**: class II obesity (obese)
- **>40**: class III obesity (morbidly obese)

Malnutrition (undernutrition)
This is an imbalanced nutritional status resulting from insufficient intake of nutrients to meet normal physiological requirements. It can be caused by inadequate access to nutrients or an end-stage sign of a chronic disease process (e.g. cancer). It is more common in the elderly population. Signs of malnutrition include:
- anaemia
- reduced muscle and/or fat mass
- oedema and/or ascites
- postural hypotension
- dermatitis and loss of hair

> **Clinical insight**
>
> A body surface area (BSA) is occasionally required to calculate insensible fluid losses or when prescribing certain medications. A useful calculation is:
>
> $$BSA\,(M^2) = \sqrt{\frac{height\,(cm) \times weight\,(kg)}{3600\,(cm\,kg/m^4)}}$$

> **Clinical insight**
>
> The following are the consequences of malnutrition: impaired immune response, reduced muscle strength and activity, loss of temperature regulation, impaired wound healing, impaired salt and fluid regulation, impaired menstrual regulation, growth failure and impaired psychosocial function. Malnutrition occurs in developed and resource-poor countries. The Malnutrition Universal Screening Tool (MUST) can be used to identify patients at nutritional risk.

Hydration
The history will give important clues to the hydration state. On clinical examination, signs of dehydration include sunken eyes, dry mucous membranes, abnormal skin turgor, delayed capillary refill, tachycardia, hypotension and a low jugular venous pressure (JVP) (**Table 2.4**).

Shock and dehydration
Shock is a state of significantly reduced systemic tissue perfusion, resulting in decreased oxygen and nutrient delivery

	Dehydration	Shock
Consciousness	Altered response	Decreased
Skin	Colour unchanged Reduced turgor	Mottled and/or pale
Cardiac	Normal peripheral pulses Normal capillary refill time Normal BP Tachycardia Tachypnoea	Weak peripheral pulses Prolonged capillary refill time Hypotension Tachycardia Tachypnoea
Extremities	Warm extremities	Cold and/or clammy
Eyes	Sunken	
Membranes	Dry or mucous	

Table 2.4 Signs of dehydration and shock

Clinical insight

Clinical staging for HIV/AIDS is a critical tool for tracking and monitoring the HIV epidemic while enabling clinicians to better treat patients, without the need for CD4 counts. The criteria are:

- primary HIV infection (i.e. asymptomatic)
- clinical stage 1 (i.e. asymptomatic with generalised lymphadenopathy)
- clinical stage 2 (e.g. moderate weight loss, herpes zoster)
- clinical stage 3 (e.g. severe unexplained weight loss, persistent oral candidiasis)
- clinical stage 4 (e.g. recurrent bacterial pneumonia, Kaposi's sarcoma)

to the tissues. Major classes of shock (and their causes) include the following:

- **Cardiogenic shock:** arrhythmias, cardiomyopathies, mechanical disturbance
- **Hypovolaemic shock:** fluid loss (e.g. diarrhoea, haemorrhage)
- **Distributive shock:** septic, anaphylactic, neurogenic
- **Combined:** a combination of the above

Dehydration (total body fluid loss) is distinctly different from shock but can cause shock.

2.6 The hands

Simultaneously inspect and palpate the hands and nails for signs of disease (**Table 2.5**). A musculoskeletal examination of the hands is described in Chapter 10.

General inspection of the hands

Inspect palmar and dorsal surfaces for deformity, colour, lesions, joint swelling and muscle wasting.

General	Skin turgor Tremor	Tar staining
Gastrointestinal	Clubbing Koilonychia Leukonychia	Dupuytren's contracture Palmar erythema
Respiratory	Tremor	
Cardiovascular	Splinter haemorrhages Janeway's lesions Osler's nodes	Xanthomas Clubbing
Rheumatological	Joint swelling Rheumatoid arthritis Rheumatoid nodules Trigger finger Deformity such as boutonnière or swan- neck deformity Palmar erythema	Osteoarthritis Heberden's or Bouchard's nodes Gout Tophi Systemic sclerosis: Sclerodactyly Telangiectasia
Dermatology	Pitting Onycholysis and onychomycosis (signs of fungal nail infection)	
Neurology	Small muscle wasting	
Thyroid	Clubbing	Palmar erythema

Table 2.5 Inspection of the hand

The palms

Palmar erythema (blotchy redness of the palms) can be a normal finding, but it is also associated with a number of conditions, e.g. pregnancy, liver disease. **Pallor** in the palmar creases indicates anaemia. **Janeway's lesions** (erythematous lesions on palms and/or soles caused by septic emboli) and **Osler's nodes** (painful, erythematous nodules caused by immune complexes) are both indicative of infective endocarditis. **Dupuytren's contracture** is a fixed flexion disorder of the palmar tendons (usually fourth and fifth digits), which is genetically inherited but can be associated with alcoholic liver disease.

The nails

Clubbing (**Figure 2.2**) is the loss of the angle between the nail bed and the nail with increased fluctuation of the nail bed. **Splinter haemorrhages** (nail-bed petechiae) are found in infective endocarditis. **Koilonychia** (spooning of the nails) is found in anaemia. **Leukonychia** (whitening of the nail bed) is found in hypoalbuminaemia.

Clubbing

This is characterised by bulbous enlargement of the fingers and/or toes (**Figure 2.2**). It is usually painless and bilateral. Although the exact cause of clubbing is unknown, it is thought to be due to hypervascularity in the nail bed. There are many conditions that are known to be associated with clubbing (**Table 2.6**), of which pulmonary disease is the most common (75%).

To assess for clubbing:

- observe the nail bed at eye level and try to note the curvature of the nail
- observe from above and try to observe soft-tissue swelling (drumstick appearance) seen in late clubbing
- place both forefinger nails together (see **Figure 2.2**); if there is a diamond-shaped 'window' between them, there is no clubbing
- feel the nail bed using your index fingers; if the nail bed moves then it is fluctuant

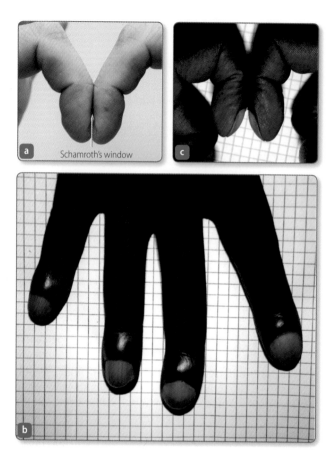

Figure 2.2 The stages and assessment of finger clubbing: (a) normal nail angle, (b, c) clubbing present.

The subcutaneous tissues

Tophi and **xanthomas** are both nodules found in the subcutaneous tissues. White tophi are urate crystals found in gout and yellow xanthomas are lipid nodules found in hyperlipidaemia.

Gastrointestinal	Cirrhosis Neoplasm Inflammatory bowel disease Malabsorption Chronic gastrointestinal infection
Cardiac	Cyanotic congenital heart disease Atrial myxoma (benign tumour) Subacute bacterial endocarditis Cor pulmonale
Respiratory	Infectious, e.g. bronchiectasis Neoplasm Idiopathic: fibrosing alveolitis Occupational: asbestosis, mesothelioma Other: pulmonary sarcoidosis, pulmonary arteriovenous malformation.
Other	Familial clubbing Hyperthyroidism Thalassaemia Pregnancy Chronic pyelonephritis or osteomyelitis

Table 2.6 Causes of clubbing

Tremor or flap

Ask the patient to stretch his or her arms out in front of them. A fine tremor can sometimes be seen only if a sheet of paper is placed on the hands. Common causes of tremor include:

- anxiety
- essential tremor
- thyrotoxicosis
- Parkinson's disease
- physiological tremor
- heavy metal poisoning, e.g. mercury, thallium

Ask the patient to hyperextend the wrists (**Figure 2.3**) and hold this position for a minimum of **15 seconds** to establish the absence or presence of asterixis. **Asterixis** is a repetitive, jerky tremor found only in severe diseases such as ventilator failure (CO_2 retention), hepatic encephalopathy, renal failure and heart failure.

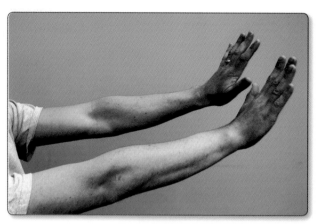

Figure 2.3 Hand position for testing for asterixis.

2.7 The neck

Inspect the neck anteriorly and laterally for changes in the skin, scars, swellings and any arterial and/or venous pulsation. Palpate the neck from behind with the patient sitting up (**Figure 2.4a**). Examine the thyroid if appropriate (Chapter 12).

Lymph nodes

Examination of the lymph nodes involves inspection and palpation. Palpation is performed using a circular motion of the three middle finger tips. There are many regions that are not accessible to examination (e.g. mesenteric nodes). Examination for **lymphadenopathy** (enlarged lymph nodes) is commonly performed in three areas:

- cervical, including supraclavicular
- axillae
- inguinal

Start with inspection and then palpate the region. Any lymphadenopathy can be described using the SSS CCC FFF TTT mnemonic (**Table 2.7**).

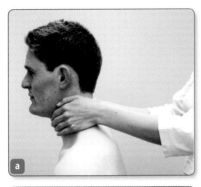

Figure 2.4 (a) Palpating the neck. (b) Cervical lymph nodes: ①, parotid nodes; ②, preauricular nodes; ③, occipital nodes; ④, mastoid nodes; ⑤, jugulodigastric node (upper deep cervical group); ⑥, submandibular gland; ⑦, submandibular nodes; ⑧, submental nodes; ⑨, internal jugular vein; ⑩, juguloomohyoid nodes (lower deep cervical group) ⑪, sternocleidomastoid; ⑫, supraclavicular nodes; ⑬ axillary vein becoming the subclavian vein proximally.

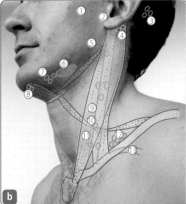

Cervical lymph node palpation

1. Position the patient in an upright, seated position.
2. Stand behind the patient (**Figure 2.4a**) as for thyroid palpation
3. Using the fingertips, systematically palpate all the regions for lymphadenopathy (**Figure 2.4b**)

Axillary lymph node palpation

1. Position the patient comfortably in an upright, seated position with the axillae exposed

S	**Site**	Describe in relation to fixed anatomical landmarks
S	**Size**	Measure the size of the lesion (with a tape measure)
S	**Shape**	Use objects to describe it, e.g. egg, golf ball, coin
C	**Colour**	What colour is the lesion?
C	**Consistency**	Soft or hard
C	**Contour**	Regular or irregular
F	**Fixed**	Mobile or fixed to the tissues around it?
F	**Fluctuant**	Fluctuant if wavelike motion when palpated.
F	**Fluid thrill**	Can a thrill be established on percussing the lesion?
T	**Temperature**	Hot?
T	**Translucency**	Translucent on placing a pen torch on the lesion
T	**Tender**	Painful to touch?

Table 2.7 Examination of 'lumps and bumps' and lesions

2. If examining the right axilla, stand on the patient's
   right and use your right
   arm to support the pa-
   tient's right arm in a 90°
   flexed and abducted position

> **Clinical insight**
>
> Distract the patient with conversation to keep their muscles relaxed.

3. Systematically palpate the axillae with the opposite hand.
   It can be useful to think of four regions forming a diamond
   (**Figure 2.5**)

Inguinal lymph node palpation
1. Position the patient lying supine
2. Palpate the horizontal and vertical groups (**Figure 6.1**).

Jugular venous pressure
The **JVP** should be assessed in the cardiovascular, respiratory
and abdominal systems and is discussed in Chapter 3.

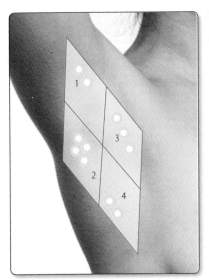

Figure 2.5 Axillary lymph nodes. ①, lateral nodes; ②, central nodes; ③, pectoral; ④, infraclavicular.

2.8 The face and mouth

The face

Inspect the face for signs of skin disease, deformity, asymmetry, lumps and characteristic facies (e.g. moon face of Cushing's syndrome). Inspect and palpate the parotid glands, which can be swollen acutely in mumps and chronically in alcohol abuse. A unilateral parotid swelling can be caused by parotitis, duct obstruction or tumour. Perform a cranial nerve (Chapter 9) and ENT examination (see below). Palpate and percuss the sinuses for evidence of tenderness (indicating sinusitis).

The mouth

Examine each part of the mouth systematically:

- **Perioral region**: look for angular stomatitis: red inflammation at the corners of the mouth caused by folate, vitamin B_{12} and iron deficiency
- **The tongue**: identify any growths or ulcers. A blue tongue suggests central cyanosis. A smooth tongue is found in iron,

folate and vitamin B_{12} deficiency. Differentiate thrush infection from benign furring of the tongue

- **The teeth**: caries can be a source of local and systemic infection. Gingivitis is inflammation of the gums often caused by chronic plaque accumulation. Gum hypertrophy is found in phenytoin treatment
- **The buccal regions:** evidence of ulcers or inflammation
- **The tonsils and oropharynx:** see ENT examination below

2.9 Ear, nose and throat

Ears

Inspect the pinna and behind the ear. Inspect for tags and/or sinuses around the ear. The ear canal extends from the pinna to the **tympanic membrane** and is an anteriorly facing canal. It is therefore best to inspect the canal and tympanic membrane using a pincer grip of the otoscope (**Figure 2.6**). Hold the otoscope as close to the head as possible to reduce pain in the ear due to hand movements. When examining the left ear, hold the otoscope in the left hand (vice versa for right). This frees up the opposite hand to support the pinna by gently holding the ear superiorly and posteriorly. This enables good visualisation of the tympanic membrane (**Figure 2.6b**); look for light reflex, grommets, cholesteatoma, effusion and/or inflammation.

> ### Clinical insight
>
> There are several classic odours that can help form a diagnosis:
>
> - **Halitosis**: malodorous breath found in bronchiectasis, poor dental hygiene and gingivitis
> - **Acetone** (like nail varnish remover): smell of breath in severe diabetic ketoacidosis
> - **Fetor hepaticus**: sickly sweet smell of breath found in liver failure

Nose

Inspect the external nose for obvious lesions. Check the patency of each nostril by having the patient exhale through each nostril individually. Tip the patient's head backwards and use an otoscope (**Figure 2.7a**) or a Thudicum speculum (**Figure 2.7b**) to inspect the septum for polyps or deviation, and the turbinates (**Figure 2.7c**). Foreign bodies can also often be found in children.

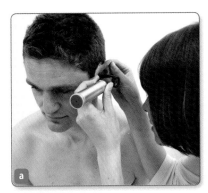

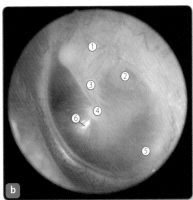

Figure 2.6 (a) Auroscopy technique; (b) View of left tympanic membrane. ①, Flaccid part of tympanic membrane; ②, projection of long process of incus; ③, handle of malleus; ④, umbo; ⑤, tense part of tympanic membrane.

If a Thudicum speculum is not available, an otoscope can be used with a larger head.

Throat

Examine the mouth as described above. Using a light source and tongue depressor (if needed), inspect the tongue, palate, uvula, tonsils and oropharynx (**Figure 2.8**). Assess the voice for change in quality, especially in respiratory disease.

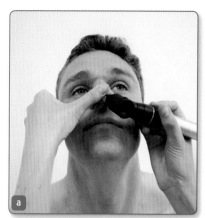

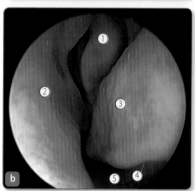

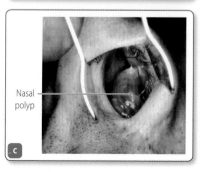

Nasal polyp

Figure 2.7 Nasal examination: (a) Otoscope, (b) Anatomy of the left nasal cavity, (c) Thudicum speculum. ①, Middle concha; ②, nasal septum; ③, inferior concha; ④, inferior meatus; ⑤, floor of nasal cavity.

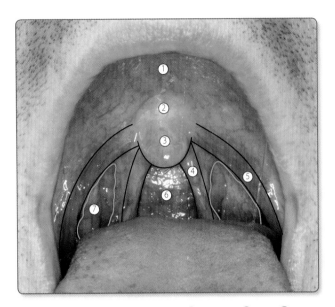

Figure 2.8 Throat inspection: ①, hard palate; ②, soft palate; ③, uvula; ④, palatopharyngeal arch; ⑤, palatoglossal arch; ⑥, oropharynx; ⑦, tonsils (green border).

2.10 The legs and feet

Peripheral vascular examination is discussed in Chapter 3.

The feet

The feet must not be obscured by socks and/or sheets. They must be inspected. Look for signs of peripheral oedema and evidence of peripheral vascular disease.

2.11 The skin and hair

The skin is the largest organ of the body and for a comprehensive discussion we suggest referring to a larger text. Examine the skin in natural light where possible. No dermatological examination is complete without examining the nails, hair and mucosa.

Skin

Perform a general inspection of the skin looking for:
- pallor, not always caused by anaemia, therefore verify at the conjunctiva
- areas of hyper- or hypopigmentation

If there are specific skin lesions then these should be both inspected and palpated in order to classify them. Note the lesion type (**Figure 2.9**), distribution (symmetrical, etc.), number, size, colour, shape, surface and edge, and the nature of the surrounding skin.

Hair

Identify areas of **alopecia** (hair loss). Women with facial hair or male pattern baldness should be investigated for polycystic ovarian syndrome, although these can often be normal variants, especially in postmenopausal women. Is the hair character normal? Are there dermatological lesions underneath the hair?

Nails

Nails often demonstrate signs of systemic disease and should be inspected as part of a thorough examination (**Table 2.8**).

'Lumps and bumps'

Inspection and palpation of 'lumps and bumps' can be helped with the mnemonic SSS CCC FFF TTT (**Table 2.7**). Auscultate the lesion for a bruit, especially if a vascular lesion is suspected. If a lesion is found palpate the local lymph nodes.

2.12 Systems examination

The history should guide the examination; therefore, once the general examination is complete, an examination of the most relevant system(s) should be undertaken.

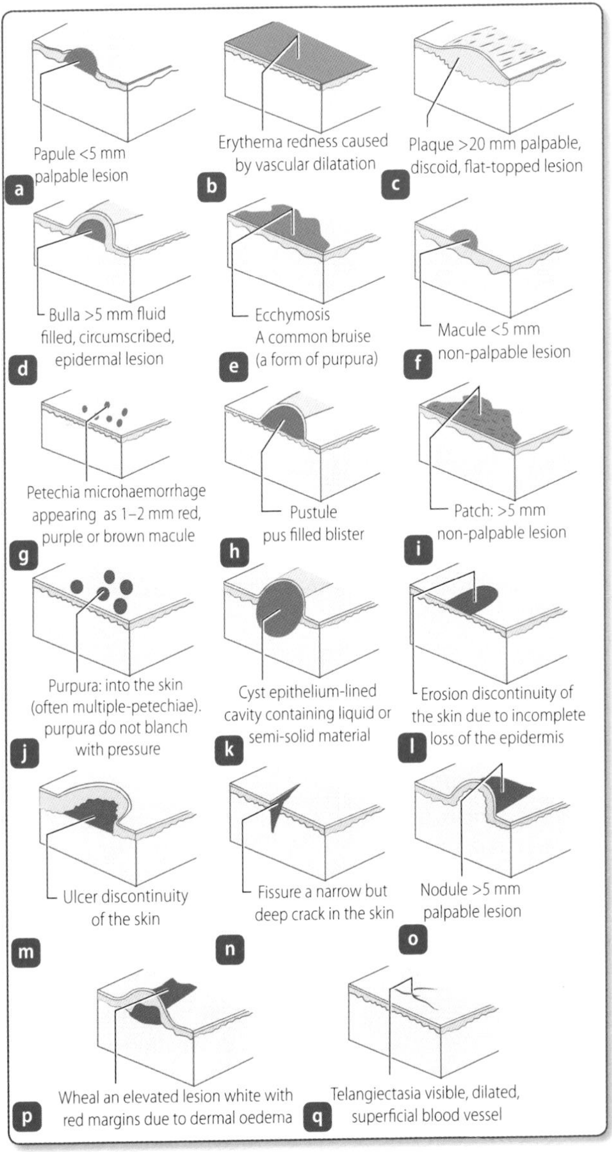

a Papule <5 mm palpable lesion

b Erythema redness caused by vascular dilatation

c Plaque >20 mm palpable, discoid, flat-topped lesion

d Bulla >5 mm fluid filled, circumscribed, epidermal lesion

e Ecchymosis A common bruise (a form of purpura)

f Macule <5 mm non-palpable lesion

g Petechia microhaemorrhage appearing as 1–2 mm red, purple or brown macule

h Pustule pus filled blister

i Patch: >5 mm non-palpable lesion

j Purpura: into the skin (often multiple-petechiae). purpura do not blanch with pressure

k Cyst epithelium-lined cavity containing liquid or semi-solid material

l Erosion discontinuity of the skin due to incomplete loss of the epidermis

m Ulcer discontinuity of the skin

n Fissure a narrow but deep crack in the skin

o Nodule >5 mm palpable lesion

p Wheal an elevated lesion white with red margins due to dermal oedema

q Telangiectasia visible, dilated, superficial blood vessel

Figure 2.9 Skin lesions.

Sign	Description	Causes
Clubbing	See **Figure 2.1**	See **Table 2.2**
Koilonychia	Spooning of the nails	Iron deficiency anaemia
Leukonychia	Whitening of the nail bed	Hypoalbuminaemia, chronic renal failure, vitiligo
Longitudinal ridging	Ridging longitudinally	Ageing, trauma, lichen planus
Transverse ridging	Horizontal ridge	Acute systemic illness (Beau's lines), eczema, psoriasis
Onycholysis	Separation of the nail from the bed	Psoriasis, trauma, nail infection, drug reaction
Onychomycosis	White or yellow discoloration with thickened, opaque nail	Fungal infection of the nail bed
Onychocryptosis (ingrown nail)	Nail growing into the paronychium or nail bed	Granuloma, incorrect nail trimming, infection
Paronychia	Inflammation of cuticle with or without pus	Acute or chronic infection
Pitting	Pinpoint or larger depressions in the nail plate	Psoriasis, alopecia, eczema
Splinter haemorrhages	Small vertical blood clots (often microemboli) under the nail	Endocarditis, psoriasis, trauma, rheumatoid arthritis

Table 2.8 Abnormalities of the nails

Cardiovascular system

The circulatory system supplies every organ and tissue in the body, so any organ can be affected by it. Ischaemic heart disease and cerebrovascular disease account for almost 25% of all global deaths. In low- and middle-income countries, the rate of cardiovascular disease is increasing rapidly due to life-style changes. In contrast, the rates of cardiovascular disease are decreasing in developed countries due to more advanced medical care.

3.1 System overview

Anatomy review

The heart

The heart consists of specialised cardiac skeletal muscle which contracts to deliver oxygen and nutrients to tissues and organs. Within the heart there are four main valves. The **atrioventricular valves** (tricuspid on the right and mitral on the left) separate the atria from the ventricles. These valves are open during ventricular relaxation (**diastole**), allowing blood to flow from the atria into the ventricles. They close during ventricular contraction (**systole**). This prevents backflow of blood from the ventricles into the atria. The closing of these valves at the start of systole can be heard as the **first heart sound** (S1).

The pulmonary and aortic valves are semilunar (bicuspid) valves that open on ventricular contraction, allowing blood to flow into the pulmonary and systemic circulation respectively (**Figure 3.1**). The **second heart sound** (S2) is heard when these semilunar valves close at the end of systole. S2 is heard as a result of two valves closing, so any abnormality in the timing will result in 'splitting' of the sound.

The peripheral vascular system

Blood is distributed to tissues by the systemic arterial circulation and then back to the heart by the venous circulation.

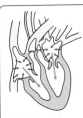

1. Atrial systole

- Atria contract, ventricles relaxed
- Tricuspid and mitral valves open
- Blood forced into ventricles
- Pulmonary and aortic valves closed

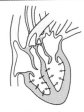

2. Early ventricular systole

- Atria relax, ventricles contract
- Tricuspid and mitral valves closed
- Pulmonary and aortic valves still closed

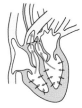

3. Late ventricular systole

- Atria relax, ventricles contract
- Tricuspid and mitral valves close
- Blood ejected from ventricles
- Pulmonary and aortic valves forced open

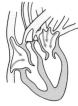

4. Early ventricular diastole

- Atria and ventricles relax
- All valves closed
- Atria begin filling with blood
- Pulmonary and aortic valves forced open

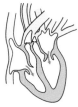

5. Late ventricular diastole

- Atria and ventricles relax
- Tricuspid and mitral valves open
- Blood starts to enter ventricles
- Pulmonary and aortic valves forced open

Figure 3.1 The cardiac cycle.

The jugular veins feed into the superior vena cava and right atrium without any intervening valves, therefore any pressure change in the right atrium will be seen in the **jugular venous pressure** (JVP).

Physiology review
The cardiac cycle

There are two main phases of the cardiac cycle: systole and diastole (**Figure 3.1**). This cycle is controlled by a sophisticated system of electrical conduction, starting in the natural pacemaker, the sinoatrial node situated in the right atrium.

> ## Clinical insight
>
> **Heart failure** is the inability of the heart to meet the body's demands for oxygen and nutrients. The primary disturbance is impairment in left ventricular function, leading to reduced stroke volume and therefore reduced cardiac output. **Pulmonary oedema** is caused by a failure of the left ventricle to remove blood from the pulmonary circulation, resulting in 'back pressure' on the lungs. Fluid therefore overflows into the interstitial lung tissue and eventually into the air-filled spaces of the lungs. **Peripheral oedema** is associated with right ventricular failure, with a similar back-pressure effect on the systemic venous return. **Congestive heart failure** is where both left- and right-sided heart failure are present in a patient; often the left-sided heart failure starts initially and causes the right heart failure.

Cardiac output

Cardiac output is the volume of blood (in millilitres) being pumped by either ventricle during 60 seconds:

$$\text{Cardiac output} = \text{Stroke volume} \times \text{Heart rate}$$

$$\text{Stroke volume} = \text{End-diastolic volume} - \text{End-systolic volume}$$

The greater the volume of blood (**preload**) entering the ventricle during diastole, the greater the volume of blood ejected out of the heart during systole. This is known as **Starling's law**.

Systemic vascular resistance The systemic vascular bed is a dynamic part of the circulatory system. Arterioles are dynamic vessels that are able to alter their diameter, thereby altering their resistance according to the body's needs. Vasoconstriction (narrowing) will increase the systemic vascular resistance (SVR). Increased SVR will raise blood pressure and reduce cardiac output.

Blood pressure

Systolic blood pressure is the peak pressure found in the arteries during ventricular contraction. **Diastolic pressure** is the minimum pressure found during ventricular relaxation:

$$\text{Blood pressure} = \text{Cardiac output} \times \text{SVR}$$

Based on this equation anything that affects either cardiac output or SVR will affect blood pressure. Physiological mechanisms are in place to maintain normal blood pressure:

- autonomic nervous system responses
- capillary shift mechanisms
- hormonal responses
- kidney and fluid balance mechanisms

3.2 Symptoms and signs

Symptoms

Take a full cardiac history (**Table 3.1**) using the mnemonic OPERATES+ (Table 1.2) for each presenting complaint or problem.

Clinical insight

Risk factors for ischaemic heart disease

- Age
- Gender (males > females)
- Family history
- Smoking
- Obesity (page 39)
- Diabetes mellitus
- Hypertension
- Hypercholesterolaemia

Chest pain

Chest pain is the most important symptom in cardiovascular disease, but can also be caused by non-cardiovascular disease (**Table 3.2**). Use the SOCRATES mnemonic (Table 1.3) to assess chest pain. The characteristics of cardiovascular chest pain will vary according to its cause. In ischaemic heart disease it tends to be a heavy or crush-

History component	Key points
Presenting complaint	Chest pain Shortness of breath Orthopnoea Nocturnal dyspnoea Oedema Palpitations Claudication Collapse Exercise intolerance
Past medical history	Cardiac disease (e.g. myocardial infarction) Murmurs Rheumatic fever
Past surgical history	Recent dental work (risk factor for infective endocarditis)
Drug history	Antihypertensives Nitrates, e.g. glyceryl trinitrate or GTN Other cardiac medications, e.g. antiarrhythmics, diuretics
Family history	Acquired cardiovascular disease Congenital heart disease Sudden death
Social history	Current or previous tobacco use Alcohol use Intravenous drug use (risk factor for infective endocarditis and deep vein thrombosis)

Table 3.1 The cardiac history

ing central chest pain, radiating to the left arm and/or jaw brought on by exertion and associated with nausea, sweating and breathlessness.

Shortness of breath

Shortness of breath (SOB), also known as **dyspnoea**, is the subjective sensation of difficulty breathing. In cardiac pathology, breathlessness can be of three main types:

1. **Exertional dyspnoea:** dyspnoea during physical exertion
2. **Orthopnoea:** dyspnoea on lying flat. Orthopnoea is highly suggestive of severe heart failure. On lying flat, the venous

Origin	Examples
Cardiovascular	Coronary artery disease, pericarditis or myocarditis, aortic dissection, valvular heart disease, pulmonary embolus
Respiratory	Acute pleural inflammation (e.g. pneumonia), infiltration of pleura (e.g. mesothelioma), pleural malignancy (including metastases), spontaneous pneumothorax, tracheal infection, pleural effusion
Musculoskeletal	Costochondritis (Tietze's syndrome), muscle sprain, rib fracture, rheumatic disease
Gastrointestinal	Oesophagitis and/or gastro-oesophageal reflux, oesophageal spasm or tear, pancreatitis, cholecystitis, perforated gastric ulcer
Other	Thymoma, lymphadenopathy, mediastinitis, herpes zoster (shingles), psychogenic

Table 3.2 Causes of chest pain

Clinical insight

New York Heart Association (NYHA) functional classification of heart failure

Class I: no limitations; ordinary physical activity does not cause fatigue, breathlessness or palpitations

Class II (mild): slight limitation of physical activity; comfortable at rest; ordinary physical activity results in fatigue, palpitation, breathlessness or angina pectoris

Class III (moderate): marked limitation of physical activity; although comfortable at rest, less than ordinary physical activity will lead to symptoms

Class IV (severe): inability to carry on any physical activity without discomfort; symptoms of cardiac failure are present even at rest

return to the heart is increased. Pulmonary oedema occurs as a consequence of pulmonary venous congestion due to poor left ventricular function

3. **Nocturnal dyspnoea:** dyspnoea wakes the patient from sleep with a gasping sensation. Often there will be pink frothy sputum after a bout of coughing

Palpitations

Palpitations are the abnormal sensation of the heart beating in the chest. Patients will often describe them as irregular, missing beats, fast, fluttery, thumping or jumping. It can be found in healthy individuals or it can be a sign of a pathological arrhythmia. In healthy people, it may be precipitated by anxiety, exercise, caffeine and alcohol, so it is important to ask about precipitating and relieving factors.

> ## Clinical insight
>
> All episodes of syncope should have lying and standing blood pressures measured along with an ECG to identify arrhythmias and/or prolonged QT interval.

Syncope

Syncope, otherwise known as **fainting**, is a sudden loss of consciousness immediately followed by a complete recovery. It is a form of non-epileptic seizure, so a seizure history is useful (page 164). Syncope is caused by an interruption in the supply of oxygen-rich blood to the brain. Cardiac causes include vasovagal syncope, arrhythmia, sinus bradycardia, heart block, ventricular tachycardia, supraventricular tachycardia, aortic stenosis and hypertrophic cardiomyopathy.

Claudication

Claudication is pain felt in the legs on walking and is relieved by rest. The pain is felt in the buttocks, thighs and/or calves. It suggests insufficient blood supply to the peripheries caused by peripheral vascular disease. Quantify the 'claudication distance', i.e. how far the patient is able to walk before the pain begins.

Signs

The key signs of cardiovascular disease are summarised in **Table 3.3**.

Hypertension and hypotension

An abnormal blood pressure (Table 2.2) can be caused by disorders of almost any system and requires a full assessment of the patient for both cardiovascular and non-cardiovascular disease.

Abnormal pulse rate

In adults, **bradycardia** is defined as <51 beats/min (bpm) and **tachycardia** as >90 bpm (Table 2.2). Exertion, pain, fever, anxiety, drugs, endocrine disease and arrhythmias cause tachycardia. Bradycardia is found during sleep and is caused by drugs, endocrine disease and arrhythmias.

Environment	Oxygen	Medications
General	Nutritional state Tendon xanthoma	Breathlessness Sweating
Vital signs	High or low BP Fever Low oxygen saturations	Tachypnoea Tachycardia
Pulses	Radial rate Abnormal rhythm	Abnormal character
Hands	Clubbing Sweating Splinter haemorrhages Palmar erythema	Nicotine staining Osler's nodes Janeway's lesions
Eyes	Corneal arcus Retinopathy	Pale conjunctiva
Face and mouth	Pallor Malar flush	Central cyanosis Poor dental hygiene
Neck	Raised jugular venous pressure Carotid pulse character	Carotid bruits Referred murmurs
Precordium	Inspect (scars, pulsations) Palpation (displaced apex, heaves, thrills)	Auscultation (abnormal heart sounds, added sounds, murmurs)
Chest	Basal crackles	Dull percussion note
Abdomen	Hepatomegaly Ascites	Aortic aneurysm
Peripheries	Radio-radio or radiofemoral delay Sacral and/or peripheral oedema	Peripheral cyanosis Absent peripheral pulses
Genitalia	Oedema	

Table 3.3 Key signs on cardiovascular examination

Crackles

Crackles, also known as crepitations, are non-musical sounds found during inspiration, caused by the reopening of collapsed or occluded alveoli. Crackles in association with other signs of cardiac disease indicate cardiogenic pulmonary oedema. Pulmonary oedema is a common and potentially fatal cause of acute respiratory distress. Causes include heart failure, fluid overload, severe hypertension, renal artery stenosis and renal disease.

Oedema

Oedema is tissue swelling caused by fluid accumulation in the interstitial space. Due to gravity, the most common sites are the lower limbs and sacrum. Heart failure and vasodilator drugs are typical causes. A raised JVP and peripheral bilateral oedema suggest right ventricular failure.

3.3 Examination of the cardiovascular system

Position the patient at 45° to the horizontal and expose the chest (maintain dignity in women with a sheet). There are 'cardiac patterns' that can lead to a clinical diagnosis (**Table 3.4**).

	Aortic stenosis	**Aortic regurgitation**	**Mitral stenosis**	**Mitral regurgitation**
Pulse	Slow rising	Collapsing	Irregularly irregular (can be in AF)	
Peripheral findings	Low blood pressure Narrow pulse pressure	Nail-bed pulsation (Quincke's sign) Carotid pulsation (Corrigan's sign)	Malar flush Signs of CCF	
JVP			Raised (late sign)	
Chest palpation	Sustained apex beat	Displaced and sustained apex beat	Tapping apex beat Left parasternal heave (late on)	Displaced and sustained apex beat
Murmur	Ejection systolic	Early diastolic (S2 may be diminished)	Mid- to end-diastolic	Pansystolic (S2 may be diminished)

Table 3.4 Cardiac patterns

Contd...

Primary site of murmur	Aortic area	Left sternal edge	Apex	Apex
Loudest heard		Expiration at lower left sternal edge with patient sat up	Lying on left side	Lying on left side
Radiation	To the carotids	Along left sternal edge	None	To the axilla
Other findings		Pistol shot femorals (Durosier's sign)	Opening mid-diastolic 'click', Loud S1	Bibasal crepitations secondary to LVF Third heart sound

AF, atrial fibrillation; CCF, congestive cardiac failure; JVP, jugular venous pressure; LVF, left ventricular failure; S2, second heart sound.

Table 3.4 *Contd...*

Vital signs

Assess the vital signs (Table 2.2). Pay particular attention to the pulse and the blood pressure.

Inspection
General Inspection
Start with a general inspection (Chapter 2), in particular looking for breathlessness and colour. Is the patient on any oxygen? If so, how much and what effect is it having (see Chapter 4)?

Inspect the chest for scars, heaves and/or pulsations. Venous collaterals on the chest or shoulders are a sign of superior vena cava, axillary or subclavian vein obstruction.

Jugular venous pulse
The JVP is a visible waveform (**Figure 3.2**) in the internal jugular vein (**Figure 3.3**) rather than a palpable pulse. Due to its anatomy, the JVP reflects the pressure in the right atrium.

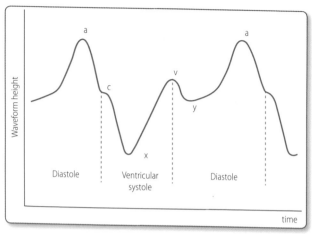

Figure 3.2 Jugular venous pressure (JVP) waveform. a, atrium contracting, tricuspid value opens; c, right ventricular contraction; x, atrium relaxing and rapid filling; v, atrium full, tricuspid valve closed; y, atrium emptying with open tricuspid.

Persistent elevation of the JVP is indicative of raised atrial pressure, so it is a reliable and early sign of right ventricular failure.

Assessing the JVP

- Position the patient with the trunk at 45° and rotate the head away from yourself
- Find the sternal angle (also known as the manubriosternal angle) and the internal jugular venous pulse (**Figure 3.4**)
- Confirm that it is the internal jugular vein (**Table 3.5**)
- Measure the peak vertical height of the waveform in centimetres (note: it is not the length of the pulsation along the vein but rather the vertical height that needs to be measured). A normal JVP is <3 cm

The hepatojugular reflex

- Ensure that the patient has no abdominal pain
- Apply firm pressure to the right upper quadrant (RUQ)
- A transient elevation in JVP for a few seconds, of approximately 2 cm, is a normal finding.

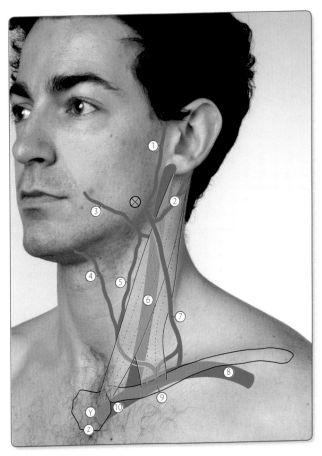

Figure 3.3 Superficial and deep veins of the neck and face: (1), Retromandibular vein; (2), posterior auricular vein; (3), facial vein; (4), anterior jugular vein; (5), communicating vein; (6), internal jugular vein; (7) external jugular vein; (8), axillary vein; (9), subclavian vein; (10), left brachiocephalic vein; ⊗, position of the mandibular angle; (Y), manubrium of sternum; (Z), sternal angle.

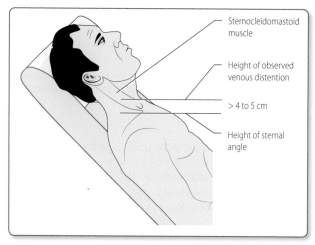

Figure 3.4 Measuring jugular venous pressure.

	JVP	Carotid pulse
Inspiration	Falls during inspiration	No effect
Waveforms	Double	Single
Pulse	Pulseless	Pulsatile
Effect of position	Varies	No effect
Abdominal pressure (hepatojugular reflex)	Rises	No effect
Compression distally	Obliterates waveform	No effect

Table 3.5 Differentiating the jugular venous pressure (JVP) from carotid pulse

Assessing the pulse
Rate and rhythm
The tips of the index and middle finger should be used to palpate the radial pulse. If the thumb is used for small, peripheral,

pulses then the clinician may inadvertently palpate their own pulse. Take the pulse rate (Table 2.2) and rhythm at the radial pulse (**Figure 3.6**). The rhythm should be regular, although inspiration quickens the pulse rate. Abnormal rhythms can be described as: **regularly irregular** (e.g. atrial flutter), **irregularly irregular** (e.g. atrial fibrillation) or **regular with ectopics** (e.g. ectopic heart beats).

Delay

While palpating the right radial pulse, simultaneously palpate the left radial pulse followed by a femoral pulse to assess for radio-radio and/or radiofemoral delay. This is indicative of stenosis affecting the arterial system proximal to the delayed pulse, e.g. **radiofemoral delay** suggests coarctation anywhere along the aorta.

Character and volume

The pulse volume and character are best assessed for abnormalities at the carotid pulse. Is the pulse of normal, reduced (weak) or increased (hyperdynamic) volume? Is there a distinctive character to the pulse (**Table 3.6**)? With your finger on the radial pulse, lift the arm to assess for a **collapsing pulse**, found in aortic regurgitation.

Pulse character	Causes
Slow rising	Aortic stenosis
Pulsus alternans	Aortic stenosis Left ventricular failure
Pulsus paradoxus	Acute asthma Cardiac tamponade Pericardial constriction
Jerky pulse	Hypertrophic cardiomyopathy
Collapsing pulse	Aortic regurgitation Arteriovenous fistula

Table 3.6 Abnormal pulse characters

Palpation

Keep the patient in a 45° position. While feeling the radial pulse, feel the temperature of the hand. Cold extremities can indicate a number of diagnoses (e.g. poor cardiac output).

Apex beat

The **apex beat** (also known as the apical impulse or point of maximal impulse) is the most distal point on the precordium (laterally and inferiorly) at which the cardiac impulse can be palpated (**Figure 3.5a**). It is caused by the heart rotating on its axis, moving forward and striking the chest wall during systole. It is normally found in the fifth intercostal space in the mid-clavicular line and can be visible on inspection. Describe the character of the apex beat. Remember its location, because this is the best place to auscultate the sounds of the mitral valve. It is not uncommon to be unable to palpate the apex beat. If it is not palpable then verify that it is not on the right side, which would indicate dextrocardia.

Lateral or inferior displacement usually indicates cardiomegaly, commonly due to cardiac dilatation. A forceful pulsation that is sustained (**heaving apex**) indicates ventricular hypertrophy (e.g. pressure overload such as hypertension). A forceful pulsation that is not sustained (**hyperdynamic apex**) indicates ventricular dilatation (e.g. volume overload). A 'tapping' apex is palpated in mitral stenosis.

> ## Clinical insight
>
> Tips for palpating the apex:
> - If the apex is difficult to palpate, ask the patient to lean forward. This will bring the heart closer to the anterior chest wall and aid palpation.
> - For a woman be sure to remove her bra. The left breast may need to be lifted in order to palpate the apex.

Heaves and thrills

Use the heel of the palm, over the left parasternal position, to palpate for heave. (**Figure 3.5b**). A parasternal heave will feel like your hand is being lifted off the chest with each systole. It is found in right ventricular hypertrophy.

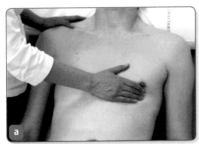

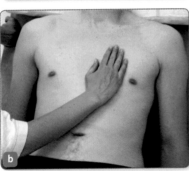

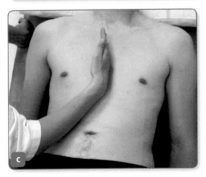

Figure 3.5 Palpation of the chest: (a) apex; (b) heave; (c) thrill.

Thrills are palpable murmurs. Place the ulnar side of your hand, or fingertips, very gently on the chest wall at each auscultation point to identify any palpable thrills (**Figure 3.5c**). They will feel like a 'buzzing' on the surface of the skin. Palpating a thrill helps classify the grade of the murmur.

Liver

Ask the patient if he or she has any pain. Palpate the liver to ascertain if it is enlarged (Figure 5.5). If it is enlarged, then percuss the upper and lower border to ensure that it is true hepatomegaly rather than the diaphragm inferiorly displacing the liver. A pulsatile liver indicates tricuspid regurgitation.

Abdominal aorta

With the patient supine, palpate between the xiphoid and umbilicus for an obvious **abdominal aortic aneurysm** (Figure 5.6). Abdominal palpation for an aortic aneurysm is not accurate for dilatation of <5 cm. Accuracy is further reduced in patients of larger body habitus.

Peripheral oedema

Inspect and palpate for peripheral oedema at the limbs and sacrum. Apply pressure for five seconds before withdrawing. If an impression of your finger remains then the oedema is pitting in nature. Note the level, i.e. how high up the body the oedema goes. Genital oedema can cause outflow obstruction.

Percussion

Percussion of the chest wall to identify cardiomegaly is rarely performed as it is an inaccurate method to establish cardiac size.

Auscultation

Resist the temptation to auscultate too early. Ensure a full and comprehensive inspection and palpation before auscultating. Using a stethoscope, the diaphragm will reveal higher-pitched sounds whereas the bell lower-pitched sounds. The bell is useful for listening over the neck for bruits and/or referred murmurs.

Heart sounds

First, find a pulse with your free hand (**Figure 3.6**). S1 is simultaneous with the pulse. Some would say that the radial pulse is inappropriate for identifying S1 due to the fractional delay. Listen over the four auscultation points (**Figure 3.7**):
- Pulmonary valve auscultation point (left edge of sternum in second intercostal space)

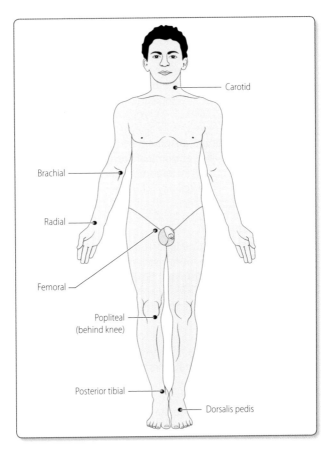

Figure 3.6 Palpation points.

- Aortic valve auscultation point (right edge of sternum in second intercostal space)
- Tricuspid valve auscultation point (left edge of sternum in fourth intercostal space)
- Mitral valve auscultation point (where the apex was palpated)

When auscultating:
- Find S1, which is simultaneous with the pulse. Then find S2. Note their character, intensity and if there is any splitting. Splitting is when the valves can be heard independently closing giving the impression of hearing two heart sounds rather than one
- Are there any extra heart sounds (**Table 3.7**)?

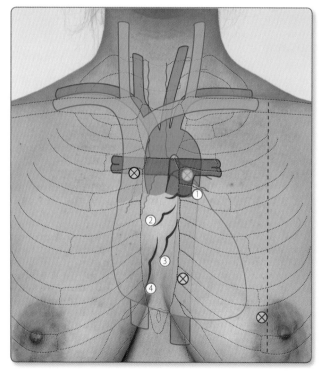

Figure 3.7 Surface markings of the heart valves and auscultation points: ①, pulmonary valve; ②, aortic valve; ③, bicuspid (mitral) valve; ④, tricuspid valve; ⊗, aortic valve auscultation point; ⊗, pulmonary valve auscultation point; ⊗, tricuspid valve auscultation point; ⊗, mitral valve auscultation point.

- Is there a murmur present? If so, describe it including the grade (**Table 3.8**)
- Is there a pericardial friction rub (characteristic of pericarditis)?
- Use the bell of the stethoscope to re-auscultate the mitral and tricuspid auscultation points for low-pitched murmurs

Describing a murmur This is any sound of vascular origin. Heart murmurs are abnormal sounds that are produced by blood

Heart sound	Physiology	Causes
Splitting of first heart sound (S1)	Non-simultaneous valve closure	Physiological (i.e. normal) Right bundle-branch block
Third heart sound (S3): ventricular gallop	Rapid ventricular filling in early diastole	Normal in children, athletes and fever Heart failure or mitral regurgitation
Fourth heart sound (S4): atrial gallop	Reduced compliance or increased stiffness of the ventricular myocardium	Never physiological Hypertension, hypertrophic cardiomyopathy, left ventricular hypertrophy
Opening snap	High left atrial pressure, forcing open stenotic valve	Mitral stenosis
Ejection click	High-pressure ventricle, forcing open stenotic valve	Aortic stenosis, pulmonary stenosis
Mid-systolic click	Prolapse of the mitral valve into the left atrium	Mitral regurgitation
Metallic valve sound	Metallic valve	Valve replacement surgery
Pericardial knock	Loss of pericardial elasticity	Pericarditis
Pericardial friction rub	Inflamed pericardial membranes	Pericarditis

Table 3.7 Extra heart sounds

Grade	Systolic murmur	Diastolic murmur
I	Very quiet (barely audible)	Very quiet (barely audible)
II	Quiet	Quiet
III	Loud (heard all over precordium)	Loud
IV	Loud with a thrill present	Very loud
V	Very loud, with a thrill	
VI	Very loud, with a thrill. Audible with stethoscope 1 cm above chest wall	

Table 3.8 Grades of systolic heart murmurs

moving through the heart or its valves. A heart murmur can help lead a clinician to a diagnosis (**Table 3.9**) and should be described accurately for the following:

- **Site:** where is it heard the loudest (see **Figure 3.7**)?
- **Timing:** systolic, diastolic or continuous (**Figure 3.8**)?
- **Grade/intensity:** the 'volume' of the murmur (**Table 3.8**)
- **Pitch:** high (high pressure gradient) or low?
- **Radiation:** heard in any other precordial auscultation points? Does it radiate to non-precordial auscultation points (carotid, axilla, left clavicle or back)?
- **Change with inspiration/posture:** any change with inspiration or expiration, or when in the left lateral or seated position?

Special auscultation techniques

- Inspiration (asking the patient to 'Take a deep breath and hold it') will increase the loudness of right-sided murmurs. Expiration (asking the patient to 'Take a deep breath, breathe out and hold it') will increase the loudness of left-sided murmurs

Clinical insight

Deciding whether a murmur is pansystolic or ejection systolic is difficult. Imagine that you can 'feel' the murmur. If it is possible to imagine 'putting your finger' between the murmur and S2 then the murmur is an ejection systolic murmur. If there is no pause and the murmur goes all the way to S2 or even obliterates it, then it is pansystolic in nature.

Auscultation point	Murmur	Diagnosis
Aortic valves	Ejection systolic	Aortic stenosis
	Pansystolic or continuous	Venous hum
Pulmonary valve	Ejection systolic	Pulmonary stenosis Aortic stenosis Innocent murmur
	Diastolic	Pulmonary regurgitation
Tricuspid valve	Pansystolic	Ventricular septal defect
	Mid diastolic	Tricuspid regurgitation
	Early diastolic (patient inhaling)	Tricuspid stenosis Aortic regurgitation
Bicuspid valve	Pansystolic	Mitral regurgitation Ventricular septal defect
	Ejection systolic	Aortic stenosis
	Mid diastolic	Mitral stenosis
	Late systolic	Mitral valve prolapse

Table 3.9 Murmurs heard at auscultation points and relative diagnosis

- Move the patient into the left lateral position. Listen over the mitral auscultation point (**Figure 3.7**) and axilla with the bell of the stethoscope, in both inspiration and expiration. A mitral stenosis murmur will be louder in this position on expiration
- Sit the patient upright and forward. Listen over the aortic auscultation point with the diaphragm of the stethoscope. Aortic regurgitation will be louder in this position on expiration

Chest
Listen over the lung fields of the back (Figure 4.4). Crepitations or crackles at the lung bases can indicate pulmonary oedema.

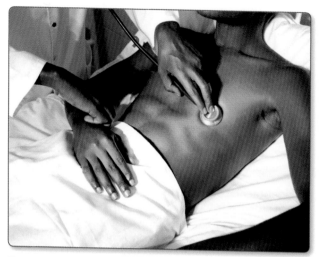

Figure 3.8 Auscultation at the apex: using the diaphragm with simultaneous radial palpation to identify S1.

Ophthalmoscopy
Ophthalmoscopy (Chapter 9) should be performed to identify signs of hypertensive or diabetic eye disease or Roth's spots in infective endocarditis.

3.4 Examination of the peripheral vascular system

General examination
Inspection
Compare the limbs for differences in colour, skin quality, rashes, hair coverage, vasculature and nutrition (muscle bulk).

Palpation
Assess the temperature of the limbs with the back of your hand, looking for areas of change. Verify the distal capillary refill time in all four limbs.

Peripheral pulses

Using your index and middle finger, palpate the major pulse points on both the right and the left side (**Figure 3.5**). Start distally, if the distal pulse is present there is no need to move to more proximal pulses. The thumb can be used on large vessels (e.g. carotid, femoral and brachial).

Calf

Palpate the calf for heat and tenderness, which could be found with a **deep vein thrombosis** (DVT). Feel for tenderness over the femoral vein, which is found medial to the femoral pulse.

Ankle–brachial pressure index

The ankle–brachial pressure index (ABPI) is a simple and cheap method to assess for arterial occlusive disease of the lower limb. The patient should rest for 10–15 min before this is undertaken. With the patient supine, use a sphygmomanometer cuff and a Doppler meter to measure the systolic pressure at the brachial artery and ankle (dorsalis pedis or posterior tibial artery). Repeat for the contralateral limb.

$$ABPI = \frac{\text{Ankle systolic pressure}}{\text{Brachial systolic pressure}}$$

ABPI values

- **>1.3:** suggests hardening of vessels (e.g. calcification)
- **0.9–1.3:** normal
- **0.4–0.9:** a degree of occlusive arterial disease, often associated with claudication
- **<0.4:** multi-level occlusive arterial disease

Auscultation

Auscultate over the major vessels (carotid, abdominal aorta, renal and femoral arteries) for arterial bruits. **Bruits** indicate turbulent blood flow and may be audible over stenosed arteries.

Varicose veins

Inspection

Inspect for varicose veins with the patient in a standing position. Varicose veins are visible, dilated, tortuous veins. They are caused by incompetent valves allowing backflow of blood from the deep veins. Note any changes to the surrounding skin and tissues.

> ## Clinical insight
>
> **Six Ps of arterial insufficiency**
>
> Acute arterial insufficiency will present with a limb that is/has:
>
> P – painful
>
> P – pulseless
>
> P – paraesthesia
>
> P – pale
>
> P – perishingly cold
>
> P – paralysed

Palpation

Are the veins hard, suggesting a thrombus within? Ask the patient to cough and assess whether pulsation is present, which would suggest valvular incompetence at the long saphenous vein in the groin.

Trendelenburg's test

Trendelenburg's test is used to assess the competency of the valves in the superficial and deep veins of the lower limbs. With the patient supine and the hip and knee flexed (i.e. leg above heart level), apply a tourniquet around the thigh. The pressure in the tourniquet should be sufficient to occlude the superficial veins but not the deep veins. Ask the patient to stand. A normal response would be filling of the superficial veins over 3–5 seconds. A more rapid filling suggests incompetence of the valves in the deep communicating veins. If there is no rapid filling, wait 20–30 seconds and release the tourniquet. If there is rapid filling of the veins, there is valve incompetence in the superficial veins. This is not to be confused with Trendelenburg's test for assessing the abductor muscles of the hip (page 238).

To finish
Mid-calf diameter
Measure the circumference of the calf at a fixed distance from the medial malleolus. Compare the circumference between the two limbs.

3.5 Common investigations

Common cardiovascular investigations include:

- **Blood tests**: creatine kinase or cardiac troponins (raised in angina and MI); lipids (atherosclerosis risk); C-reactive protein, ESR or ferritin (indicate inflammation)
- **12-lead electrocardiography**: to identify abnormalities of ventricular rate, rhythm, cardiac axis, atrial activity and/or conduction intervals
- **Echocardiography**: ultrasound visualisation of cardiac chambers, walls and valves and their movement, and estimation of blood flow and cardiac output
- **BP monitoring**
- **Chest radiography**: posterior-anterior film to assess for cardiomegaly and/or pulmonary oedema. Postoperatively to identify thoracic complications
- **Carotid ultrasonography**: to assess for atherosclerosis and risk of cerebrovascular events
- **Coronary angiography:** ('catheterisation'): to view coronary circulation and to assess coronary artery narrowing and cardiac chamber size, muscle contraction and valve function

3.6 System summary

A summary of the cardiovascular examination is given in **Table 3.10**.

Preparation	Wash hands; ensure privacy; introduce self and explain examination; gain consent for examination; offer a chaperone Position patient (45° angle) and expose area being examined
Vital signs	Temperature; pulse rate; respiratory rate; oxygen saturation (what is their inspired oxygen?); blood pressure in both arms; capillary refill time
Inspection	Inspection of environment; general comfort and breathing pattern Inspection of hands and face; inspection of chest (scars, symmetry, deformity, visible pulsation); jugular venous pressure (including hepatojugular reflex)
Palpation	Pulse rhythm (both radials for radio-radio delay) Femoral pulse with right radial for radiofemoral delay Pulse character and volume (carotid) Precordial palpation for: apex position and nature, heave or thrill Peripheral oedema Palpate liver
Percussion	Liver
Auscultation	Auscultate four areas of chest while palpating a pulse (listen with bell and diaphragm) Auscultate with patient in left lateral and forward seated position Comment on any murmur or added sounds Auscultate over carotids Lung bases (simultaneously checking for sacral oedema)
Finish	Lying and standing blood pressure; peripheral pulses Thank and cover the patient, and wash your hands

Table 3.10 Examination of the cardiovascular system: a summary

Respiratory system

Lower respiratory tract infections, respiratory tract cancers, chronic lung disease and tuberculosis (TB) are among the top 10 causes of death worldwide. Lifestyle issues such as smoking, occupation and obesity can contribute to respiratory disease. Examination of the respiratory system may be very difficult to interpret, especially in young children or in the early stages of some chronic diseases. A good focused history and examination are therefore essential for a correct diagnosis.

4.1 System overview

Anatomy review

The **respiratory tract** extends from the oral cavity through to the alveoli. Chest surface anatomy is shown in **Figure 4.1**.

Upper respiratory tract

The upper airway includes the nasal cavity, mouth, larynx and pharynx (**Figure 2.8**).

Lower respiratory tract

The **trachea** extends from the cricoid cartilage (at the level of the sixth cervical vertebra, C6) to its bifurcation (at the level of the fourth thoracic vertebra, T4). The **bronchial tree** subsequently consists of up to 23 further divisions of the airway. The **left lung** is divided into upper and lower lobes and is slightly smaller than the right lung, which is divided into upper, middle and lower lobes.

Blood supply

The lungs have two blood supplies: the pulmonary circulation provides deoxygenated blood from the right side of the heart ready for gas exchange, and the bronchial circulation provides oxygenated blood for the lung tissue itself.

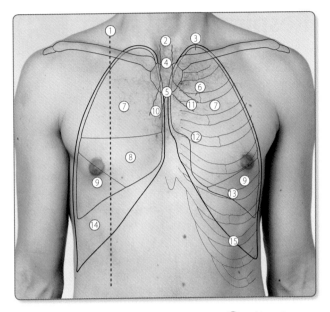

Figure 4.1 Anterior surface markings of lung and pleura: (1), Midclavicular line; (2), trachea; (3), lung apex; (4), sternal notch; (5), sternal angle/plane and tracheal bifurcation; (6), 2nd costal cartilage; (7), superior lobe of lung; (8), middle lobe of lung; (9), inferior lobe of lung; (10), right main bronchus; (11), left main bronchus; (12), 4th costal cartilage; (13), 6th rib in the midclavicular line; (14), costodiaphragmatic recess; (15), 8th costal cartilage in the midclavicular line.

Physiology review

Motor pathways

The **diaphragm**, innervated by the phrenic nerve, is the main muscle generating the negative intrathoracic pressure that produces inspiration. The **external intercostal muscles**, innervated by the intercostal nerves, T1–12, and the accessory muscles of respiration (sternocleidomastoids and scalenes) provide some additional inspiratory effort, with the latter being involved only during exercise or respiratory distress.

Control of breathing

A group of **respiratory centres** found within the brain stem control breathing subconsciously. **Peripheral** and **central chemoreceptors** monitor arterial carbon dioxide levels and pH, and act on the medullary respiratory centre to regulate minute ventilation. Peripheral chemoreceptors of the aortic and carotid bodies stimulate respiration when there is low arterial oxygen.

Gas exchange

The lungs have two functions: **oxygenation** and **ventilation** (CO_2 exchange). Oxygen is transported from the alveoli to the capillaries; 98% is bound to haemoglobin and the remainder dissolves in the plasma. In the other direction, 10% of CO_2 is dissolved in the plasma, 30% is bound to haemoglobin (carboxyhaemoglobin) and the rest is transported as carbonate (HCO_3^-).

> ### Clinical insight
>
> In patients with type II respiratory failure, the persistently elevated CO_2 levels result in reduced sensitivity of central chemoreceptors. Respiration is therefore more dependent on the peripheral chemoreceptor response to low PaO_2. Starting oxygen therapy too high in these patients decreases their respiratory drive, causing respiratory suppression. This will ultimately cause increased $PaCO_2$, further respiratory acidosis and could lead to death.

Clinically, it is important to always divide these two processes. Respiratory failure is by definition inadequate gas exchange:

- **Type I respiratory failure** is hypoxia (arterial partial pressure of oxygen or PaO_2 <8 kPa or <60 mmHg) with normocapnia (normal arterial partial pressure of carbon dioxide or $PaCO_2$)
- **Type II respiratory failure** is hypoxia with hypercapnia ($PaCO_2$ >6 kPa). If a patient is acidotic due to a high $PaCO_2$, then increasing oxygen delivery will not assist the patient and could make the situation worse

4.2 Symptoms and signs

Take a full respiratory history (**Table 4.1**) using the mnemonic OPERATES+ (Table 1.2) for each presenting complaint or problem.

History component	Key points
Presenting complaint	Cough Shortness of breath Wheeze Sputum (colour, volume) Haemoptysis (blood) Chest pain
Past medical history	Pneumonia Tuberculosis
Past surgical history	Asthma Chronic obstructive pulmonary disease and infectious exacerbations
Drug history	Inhalers (many patients will not view these as a medication) Immunisation history (in children or when clinically relevant)
Family history	Lung cancer Atopy (e.g. eczema, allergic rhinitis and/or asthma) Genetic conditions (e.g. cystic fibrosis, Alpha-1-antitrypsin deficiency) Rheumatological conditions
Social history	Current or previous tobacco use (quantify it in pack-years) Occupational exposure to lung toxins Exposure to pets can cause a variety of lung disease (e.g. asthma from cat fur)

Table 4.1 The respiratory history

Symptoms
Cough
Cough is caused by an irritation to the airways caused by infection, inflammation, a foreign body or a tumour. When the irritation occurs lower down in the airways, it may be associated with the production of sputum.

A cough should be classified as follows:

- **Duration**: acute (<3 weeks), subacute (3–8 weeks) or chronic (>8 weeks) (**Table 4.2**)
- **Character**: e.g. barking cough in a child with croup

Onset	Secondary to infection	Non-infectious
Acute (<3 weeks)	Viral upper respiratory tract infections (e.g. the common cold) Bacterial infections (e.g. pneumonia) Sinusitis Acute bronchitis	Inhaled foreign body Acute extrinsic allergic alveolitis Inhalation of irritants (e.g. fumes)
Subacute (3–8 weeks) and chronic (>8 weeks)	Postnasal drip after a viral upper respiratory tract infection Tuberculosis Superadded infection in chronic lung conditions (e.g. cystic fibrosis)	Poorly controlled asthma Lung cancer Bronchiectasis (can have infective exacerbations) COPD (can have infective exacerbations) Parenchymal lung disease Chronic sinusitis Gastro-oesophageal reflux disease Allergic rhinitis Drugs (e.g. ACE inhibitors) Habit cough

ACE, angiotensin-converting enzyme; COPD, chronic obstructive pulmonary disease.

Table 4.2 Causes of cough

- **Quality**: productive (sputum) or non-productive (dry)
- **Timing**: nocturnal, daytime or mixed

Shortness of breath (dyspnoea)

Dyspnoea is the sensation of breathlessness perceived by the patient. It is often exacerbated by exertion, so the patient's level of exercise tolerance should always be determined.

Clinical insight

A cough associated with any one of the following 'red-flag' features should always prompt further investigation including a chest radiograph:

- copious chronic sputum production
- haemoptysis
- systemic symptoms (fever, sweats, weight loss)
- chest pain
- significant dyspnoea

Dyspnoea can be caused by non-respiratory (e.g. cardiac, anaemia, ascites) or respiratory (**Table 4.3**) pathology. Specific types of dyspnoea include:

- **orthopnoea** – dyspnoea on lying flat, relieved by sitting upright
- **paroxysmal nocturnal dyspnoea** – breathlessness causing the patient to wake at night

Sputum

Sputum is excess mucus coughed up (expectorated) from the lower airways and must be differentiated from saliva. Defining its appearance (colour, consistency and presence of blood) can help differentiate the underlying disease, e.g. the expectorated sputum in pulmonary oedema is usually watery, pink and frothy.

Haemoptysis

Haemoptysis is blood that has been coughed up, and must be distinguished from a gastrointestinal bleed or bleeding from

Onset	Causes
Acute (seconds to minutes)	Pneumothorax Pulmonary embolism Inhaled foreign body
Subacute (hours to days)	Acute exacerbation of asthma Pneumonia Exacerbation of COPD
Chronic (weeks to years)	COPD Pleural effusion Respiratory neuromuscular disorders (e.g. Guillain–Barré syndrome) Pulmonary fibrotic disorders Pulmonary tuberculosis Pulmonary carcinoma Bronchiectasis Pulmonary sarcoidosis Chest wall deformities (e.g. kyphoscoliosis)
COPD, chronic obstructive pulmonary disease.	

Table 4.3 Respiratory causes of dyspnoea common or important examples

the nasal or oral cavities. Haemoptysis is always a 'red-flag' symptom and must be evaluated thoroughly. Causes can be infectious (e.g. TB), cardiac (e.g. left ventricular failure), vascular (e.g. pulmonary embolus), oncological (e.g. bronchial carcinoma), haematological (e.g. coagulation disorders) or traumatic (e.g. foreign body).

Signs
The key signs of respiratory disease are summarised in **Table 4.4**.

Abnormal chest percussion
There are four types of percussion sound:
1. **Dull**: heart, liver, lung consolidation or collapse, spleen

General	Confusion/agitation Respiratory distress Sputum pots	Cachexia Hoarseness Stridor
Environment	Oxygen Medications	Inhalers or nebulisers Sputum pot
Vital signs	Raised respiratory rate Fever	Low oxygen saturation Tachy- or bradycardia
Hands and wrists	Temperature Clubbing Tar or nicotine staining	Asterixis Pulsus paradoxus
Face	Nasal flaring Pursed lips	Ptosis Central cyanosis
Neck	Raised jugular venous pressure Lymphadenopathy	Accessory muscle use Tracheal deviation
Chest	Deformity or scars Accessory muscle use Asymmetrical expansion Abnormal percussion note	Abnormal breath sounds Added sounds Abnormal vocal resonance
Abdomen	Depressed liver edge	
Peripheries	Peripheral cyanosis Swelling	Oedema

Table 4.4 Key signs on respiratory examination

2. **Stony dull**: pleural effusion
3. **Resonant**: found in a normal air filled lung
4. **Hyperresonant**: pneumothorax, emphysema

Bronchial breathing

Bronchial breathing has a hollow or blowing quality (high pitched) on auscultation which occurs when there is consolidation or localised fibrosis, or it can be heard above a pleural effusion.

Crackles

Crackles (also known as crepitations) are non-musical sounds found during inspiration, caused by the reopening of collapsed or occluded alveoli. Determine the timing and quality of the crackles:

- **Early inspiratory crackles**: small airway disease (e.g. bronchiolitis in infants)
- **Late inspiratory crackles**: pulmonary oedema, pulmonary fibrosis, infectious exacerbation of chronic obstructive pulmonary disease (COPD), pneumonia
- **Inspiratory and expiratory crackles**: bronchiectasis
- **Coarse crackles**: these are referred sounds from larger airways due to excess secretions, e.g. in bronchiectasis. Altered on airway clearing, i.e. coughing

Reduced chest expansion

If expansion is reduced bilaterally, this suggests generalised fibrotic lung disease, spinal or chest wall deformity, or a significant air trapping disease such as COPD. If expansion is reduced unilaterally, this suggests disease on that side of the lung; it includes localised fibrosis, effusion, pneumothorax, consolidation and collapse.

Reduced breath sounds

Breath sounds are reduced on auscultation if there is a pleural effusion, pleural thickening, pneumothorax (due to decreased conduction), bronchial obstruction, asthma or COPD.

Rub

Rubs are squeaking or creaking sounds found on auscultation. They are caused by friction during the rubbing of two pleural layers that are inflamed. They are best heard with the stethoscope diaphragm at the end of inspiration. A rub suggests effusion, pneumonia or pulmonary infarction.

Silent chest

A silent chest is when there are no breath sounds on auscultation. This is found in life-threatening asthma. No breath sounds are heard due to minimal or no movement of air in the small airways.

Wheeze and stridor

It is important to clarify whether an extra respiratory noise is inspiratory (**stridor**) or expiratory (**wheeze**).

Wheeze results from constriction of the bronchioles and may be:

- **monophonic** (a single note), indicating partial obstruction of one airway, e.g. a foreign body or tumour
- **polyphonic** (multiple notes), indicating widespread airway obstruction in asthma, COPD and bronchiolitis in babies

Stridor is a harsh inspiratory sound indicating narrowing of the larynx, trachea or main bronchi. It is a serious finding and requires urgent investigation and management. Although classically inspiratory it can be heard in expiration in severe disease. The cause of stridor can be infectious (e.g. epiglottitis), environmental (e.g. inhaled foreign body), anatomical (e.g. laryngomalacia), external (e.g. mediastinal tumour) or iatrogenic (e.g. post-intubation).

4.3 Examination of the respiratory system

Start by preparing yourself for the examination: wash your hands, introduce yourself to the patient, position the patient appropriately at 45°, expose the chest and position yourself on the patient's right. Vital signs (Table 2.2) can be taken at the start or the end of the examination.

General examination

General inspection

Start by inspecting the environment for inhalers, oxygen and/or a sputum pot. Then, having adequately exposed the patient, inspect him or her to ascertain the following, specific to the respiratory system:

- Is there an adequate airway?
- Is the breathing pattern normal and what is the rate?
- Is the patient using accessory muscles of respiration?
- Is the patient pale or cyanosed?
- Is the patient cachectic?
- Is the patient comfortable or distressed?

> ## Clinical insight
>
> Central cyanosis will develop if the peripheral arterial saturation are <85% in a person with a normal haemoglobin value. This equates to a PaO_2 of 8 kPa. Remember that central cyanosis will not be obvious in a patient who is anaemic and may be exaggerated in a patient who is polycythaemic. The most common respiratory cause of central cyanosis is obstructive airway disease.

Inspect the hands for clubbing, a flapping tremor (asterixis) and/or tar staining (see Chapter 2). Look at the tongue and lips for blue discoloration due to central cyanosis. Inspect the eyes for anaemia. Assess if there is ptosis and a constricted pupil, which represents Horner's syndrome. This can be a sign of a tumour in the apex of the lung.

Oxygen

Note if the patient is on oxygen. If so, there are a number of things to ask:

1. Why is the patient on oxygen? The patient has either increased an oxygen demand (e.g. sepsis) or a reduced 'supply' (e.g. lung disease).
2. How is the oxygen being delivered (e.g. standard mask, see box opposite), and at what concentration?
3. What effect is the oxygen therapy having on the patient? The patient should be monitored with oxygen saturation and/or arterial blood gases.
4. Is there a contraindication to oxygen (e.g. type II respiratory failure, see page 87)?

Inspection of the jugular venous pressure

Inspect the neck for the jugular venous pressure (JVP) (Chapter 3). A raised JVP in respiratory disease can indicate cor pulmonale (right-sided heart failure due to lung disease) or obstruction of the superior vena cava (e.g. carcinoma of the bronchus).

Inspection of the chest

To best inspect the chest, ask the patient to sit upright and put the arms behind the neck. Inspect anteriorly and posteriorly for the following:

- scars
- venous dilatation
- abnormal chest shapes, e.g. pectus excavatum (funnel chest), pectus carinatum (pigeon chest), barrel chest (increased anteroposterior diameter), Harrison's sulcus (a groove at the lower end of the ribcage)
- spinal deformity, e.g. kyphoscoliosis
- The depth of breathing: hyperventilation and deep breathing may be associated with acidosis
- Signs of respiratory distress such as accessory muscle use

> ## Clinical insight
>
> Oxygen can be delivered via low-flow or high-flow devices. If a patient's peak inspiratory flow rate is greater than the fresh gas flow provided by the device (e.g. a simple facemask), then room air will be sucked in around the side of the mask (air entrainment) and affect the concentration of oxygen being delivered.
>
> Delivery devices include:
>
> - nasal cannulae: 1–4 litres/min (L/min); this should be humidified if >2 L/min. Rule of thumb is that 1 L/min gives an extra 4% oxygen
> - low flow:
>   - simple facemask delivers 6–12 L/min at concentration of 28–50% oxygen
>   - non-rebreathe mask (reservoir) delivers 10–15 L/min and can reach concentrations of 100% oxygen
> - high flow: specialist mask delivering >30 L/min at concentrations of up to 50% oxygen.

- Timing of inspiration and expiration: prolonged expiration indicates lower airway obstruction as in asthma or COPD
- Chest expansion: is it symmetrical?
- Audible sounds heard from the end of the bed: can a wheeze or stridor be clearly heard?
- Other patterns of breathing: are there periods of breathing cessation indicating central neurological disease, or perhaps whooping cough in a young infant?

Palpation

Trachea

To palpate the trachea (**Figure 4.2**), gently place three fingers in the midline of the neck superior to the sternal notch.

The middle finger lies on the centre of the trachea. Place the fingers either side of the middle finger on the sternocleido-mastoid tendons, and then observe to see if the distance from each tendon and the trachea is equal. If the trachea is deviated this suggests mediastinal shift or a neck lesion (**Figure 4.2**).

Apex

The normal position of the **apex** is in the fifth intercostal space, midclavicular line, palpated with the patient lying at an angle of 45°. Deviation of the apex indicates lower mediastinal shift, which is often associated with heart disease (see Chapter 3). Palpate for any heaves and/or thrills. A heave at the lower left sternal edge may indicate pulmonary hypertension causing right ventricular hypertrophy.

Clinical insight

The trachea is pulled towards lung lesions that involve collapse or fibrosis (the lung space is constricted), and pushed away from lesions that involve air and fluid collection, e.g. tension pneumothorax or a large pleural effusion (the lung space is pushed by the collections).

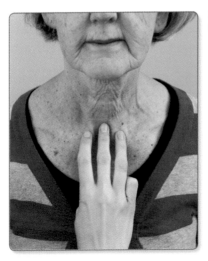

Figure 4.2 Assessing for tracheal deviation.

Lymph nodes

Palpate for cervical lymphadenopathy from behind the patient. Include palpation of the axillary region for axillary lymphadenopathy, which may be present in respiratory conditions.

Chest expansion

Feel for chest expansion (**Figure 4.3**) by using both hands to lightly grip the sides of the chest wall. Watch the movement of your thumbs on deep inspiration. In adults, this should be >5 cm and symmetrical.

Chest percussion

The method of percussion is described in Chapter 2 (Figure 2.1). Chest percussion is performed by percussing the intercostal space. Percuss the lung fields, alternating right and left, comparing each side's percussion note (**Figure 4.4**). Repeat on the back. Repeated percussion directly on to the clavicle can be painful and should be done only if necessary. If an area of abnormal resonance is found, then determine the extent by mapping out the boundary of the abnormal area.

Tactile vocal fremitus

Place the ulnar border of your hands parallel in the positions shown in **Figure 4.4**. Ask the patient to repeat the number '99' and feel the vibrations in the edge of your hand. Increased fremitus implies consolidation.

Auscultation

Ask the patient to take deep breaths through an open mouth. Breath sounds are predominantly high pitched, so use the diaphragm of your stethoscope to listen over symmetrical areas of the anterior, posterior and axillary regions of the chest wall (**Figure 4.4**). Use the bell to listen over the supraclavicular fossae. Take your time to listen to both inspiration and expiration.

Vocal resonance

Listen with your stethoscope over the areas shown in **Figure 4.4**. Ask the patient to repeat the number '99' in a low voice.

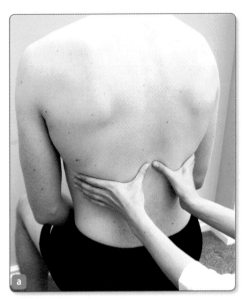

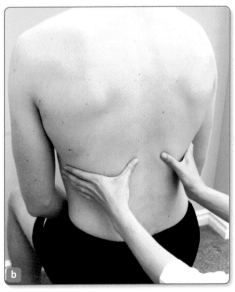

Figure 4.3
Palpation for chest expansion: (a) expiration; (b) inspiration.

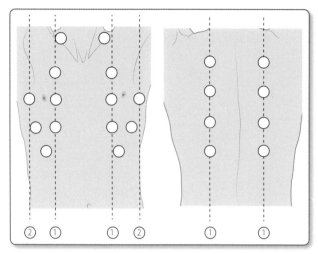

Figure 4.4 Positions on the chest wall for percussion and auscultation with anatomical landmarks. Dashed lines: ① represent midclavicular lines; ② midaxillary lines.

Vocal resonance is the sound produced by air moving from what should be an empty cavity, the lung. It is therefore altered by changes in this cavity. The resonance can be normal, diminished (e.g. pneumothorax, pleural effusion) or increased (e.g. consolidation). **Whispering pectoriloquy** is assessed by asking the patient to whisper '99'. The ability to hear vocal resonance even when the patient whispers is found in consolidation.

Vocal fremitus, vocal resonance and auscultation with a stethoscope are all effectively assessing for the same pathology, with similar signs found. It may seem unnecessary to do all three but the signs found in respiratory disease are often so subtle that it is difficult to interpret the findings on their own.

Figure 4.5 summarises some of the main lung pathologies and demonstrates how clinical examination can help differentiate between the differential diagnoses.

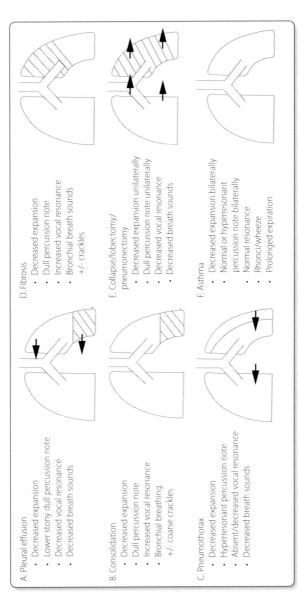

A. Pleural effusion
- Decreased expansion
- Lower stony dull percussion note
- Decreased vocal resonance
- Decreased breath sounds

B. Consolidation
- Decreased expansion
- Dull percussion note
- Increased vocal resonance
- Bronchial breathing
- +/- coarse crackles

C. Pneumothorax
- Decreased expansion
- Hyperresonant percussion note
- Absent/decreased vocal resonance
- Decreased breath sounds

D. Fibrosis
- Decreased expansion
- Dull percussion note
- Increased vocal resonance
- Bronchial breath sounds
- +/- crackles

E. Collapse/lobectomy/ pneumonectomy
- Decreased expansion unilaterally
- Dull percussion note unilaterally
- Decreased vocal resonance
- Decreased breath sounds

F. Asthma
- Decreased expansion bilaterally
- Normal or hyperresonant percussion note bilaterally
- Normal resonance
- Rhonci/wheeze
- Prolonged expiration

Figure 4.5 Summary of physical signs on respiratory examination (arrows indicate deviation of chest anatomy).

Completing the examination

To complete the examination inspect any sputum that is available. Perform a full ear, nose and throat (ENT) examination (see Chapter 2), which should include an assessment of the patient's voice. Thank and cover the patient before washing your hands. In some cases a peak flow may need to be performed (see below).

4.4 Common investigations

Common investigations of respiratory disease include:

- **Chest radiograph:** to visualise thoracic structures and lesions
- **Pulse oximetry:** to measure oxygen saturation of haemoglobin
- **Arterial blood gases:** to assess metabolic and respiratory state
- **Blood tests**: full blood count (for signs of inflammation, for abnormal cells in neoplasia or anaemia); urea and electrolytes, glucose, calcium and liver function tests (to identify causes or complications of lung disease or its treatment); C-reactive protein or erythrocyte sedimentation rate (for inflammation due to infection, inflammatory disease or neoplasia)
- **Cardiac- and pulmonary-specific blood tests**: troponin or creatine kinase (raised in ischaemic heart disease and acute pulmonary embolism, PE), D-dimers (raised during PE)
- **Virus serology and interferon gamma release assay:** (for latent TB infection)
- **Sputum culture:** to identify bacterial causes of lung infection
- **Lung function tests**: peak expiratory flow rate (reduced by airway obstruction), spirometry (differentiates obstructive and restrictive airway disease), transfer factor (i.e. CO-diffusing capacity of the lung - lower in diseases reducing the effective respiratory membrane, e.g. fibrosis, restrictive lung disease)
- **Bronchoscopy:** to identify tumours or foreign bodies, and obtain samples biopsy and culture samples
- **CT pulmonary angiography:** (CT with contrast medium) to identify pulmonary embolism and pleural disease

4.5 System summary

A summary of the respiratory examination is given in **Table 4.5**.

Preparation	Wash hands; ensure privacy; introduce self and explain examination Gain consent for examination; offer a chaperone; position patient (upright) and expose area being examined
Vital signs	Temperature; pulse rate; respiratory rate; saturation (what is their inspired oxygen?); blood pressure; capillary refill time (in children)
Inspection	Inspect environment for clues (e.g. oxygen mask, inhalers, sputum pot); general comfort and breathing pattern; nutrition assessment. Inspect hands (including tremor), face and chest (scars, symmetry, deformity); jugular venous pressure
Palpation	Tracheal position; lymph nodes in neck; chest expansion; tactile vocal fremitus Apex beat; ankle oedema
Percussion	Anterior chest and axillae; clavicles; posterior chest
Auscultation	Anterior chest; supraclavicular region (with bell); axillae; posterior chest Vocal resonance; heart (with finger on pulse)
Finish	Sputum examination. Full ear, nose and throat examination Assessment of the voice Request peak expiratory flow rate Thank and cover the patient and wash your hands

Table 4.5 Examination of the respiratory system: a summary

Gastrointestinal system

The gastrointestinal (GI) tract runs from the mouth to the anus. The symptoms and signs of GI disease are often vague and non-specific. The history remains the most important part of the consultation in combination with a thorough examination and with some system-specific features.

5.1 System overview

Anatomy review

The abdomen

The abdominal cavity is separated from the thorax by the diaphragm. For clinical descriptions, the abdomen is divided into nine regions and/or four quadrants (**Figure 5.1**).

The abdomen contains organs from most systems:

- **Gastrointestinal tract (GIT)**: oesophagus, stomach (**Figure 5.2a**), small intestine (duodenum, jejunum and ileum), large intestine (**Figure 5.2b**), rectum, anus, liver, gallbladder and exocrine pancreas
- **Cardiovascular**: abdominal aorta and branches, inferior vena cava and branches
- **Endocrine**: endocrine pancreas, adrenal glands, gonads
- **Immunological**: spleen and lymph nodes (abdominal and inguinal)
- **Urinary**: kidneys, ureters, bladder and urethra.

The abdomen is lined with a double layer of membranous tissue known as the **peritoneum.** Within the peritoneal cavity (i.e. between these two layers) is a small amount of fluid which acts as a lubricant to allow movement of the organs. The pancreas, ascending and descending colon, a portion of the duodenum and the kidneys lie behind the peritoneum and are therefore **retroperitoneal**.

The rectum and anal canal

The rectum is the terminal portion of the colon and is approximately 10–15 cm in length. The anal canal is about 5 cm in length, and its musculature forms the internal (involuntary) and external (voluntary) sphincters.

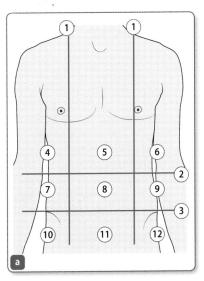

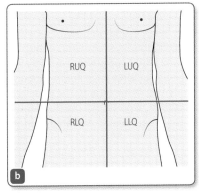

Figure 5.1 (a) Abdominal regions and (b) quadrants. ①, midclavicular line, ②, subcostal plane, ③, transtubercular plane, ④, right hypochondrium, ⑤, epigastrium, ⑥, left hypochondrium, ⑦, right lumbar/flank, ⑧, umbilical, ⑨, left lumbar/flank, ⑩, right inguinal, ⑪, pubic (hypogastrium), ⑫, left inguinal. RUQ, right upper quadrant, LUQ, left upper quadrant, RLQ, right lower quadrant, LLQ, left lower quadrant.

Physiology review
Peristalsis

Foodstuffs are moved through the GIT via organised muscle contractions known as **peristalsis**. These ensure **motility** and can be heard as bowel sounds (**borborygmi**).

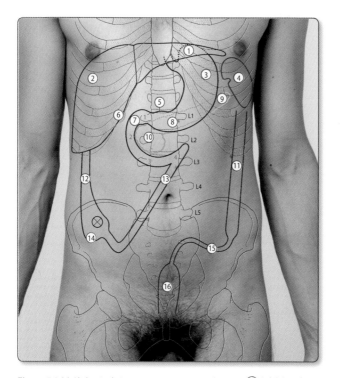

Figure 5.2 (a) Abdominal viscera an mesentery attachments: ①, left lobe of liver overlying fundus of stomach; ②, right lobe of liver; ③, stomach; ④, spleen; ⑤, pylorus; ⑥, gallbladder fundus (9th costal cartilage tip); ⑦, duodenum (four parts labelled 1–4); ⑧, neck and body of pancreas; ⑨, tail of pancreas; ⑩, head of pancreas; ⑪, descending colon; ⑫, site of ascending colon; ⑭, caecum; ⑮, attachment of sigmoid colon mesentery; ⑯, rectum; X, site of appendix attachment to caecum. *Contd...*

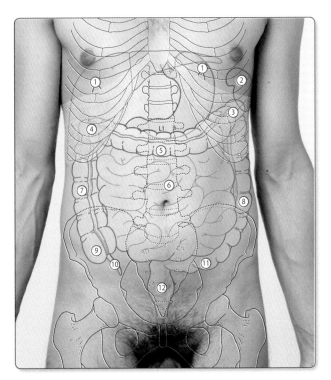

Figure 5.2 *Contd...* (b) Small and large intestine: (1), Region of costodiaphragmatic recess (white hatch); (2), spleen; (3), splenic flexure of colon; (4), hepatic flexure of colon; (5), transverse colon; (6), small intestine (ileum and jejunum); (7), ascending colon; (8), descending colon; (9), caecum; (10), appendix; (11), sigmoid colon; (12), rectum.

5.2 Symptoms and signs

Symptoms

Take a full GI history (**Table 5.1**) using the mnemonic OPERATES+ (Table 1.2) for each presenting complaint or problem.

Abdominal pain/dyspepsia

Use **the mnemonic SOCRATES** (Table 1.3) to assess abdominal pain. The location of the pain can be useful in determining a

History component	Key points
Presenting complaint	Nausea and vomiting Haematemesis Diarrhoea or constipation Dyspepsia (indigestion) Dysphagia (difficulty swallowing) Odynophagia (pain on swallowing) Change in bowel habit Rectal bleeding Jaundice Pruritis ani Loss of weight or appetite Abdominal pain, mass or swelling
Past medical history	Peptic ulcer disease, carcinoma, jaundice, hepatitis, diabetes, anaemia, blood transfusions, HIV, inflammatory bowel disease
Past surgical history	Previous abdominal or gynaecological operations Last menstrual period in women
Drug history	Analgesia and anti-inflammatory use
Family history	Bowel cancer Pancreatitis
Social history	Current or previous tobacco use (quantify it in pack-years) Alcohol use Illicit drug use (especially needle sharing) and tattoos

Table 5.1 The gastrointestinal history

cause. There are some conditions that give characteristic pain descriptions (**Table 5.2**).

Dysphagia and odynophagia

Dysphagia (difficulty swallowing) **and** **odynophagia** (painful swallowing) are common symptoms that can be caused by GI, neurological and/or ear, nose and throat (ENT) problems. Establish the onset and course of the symptoms

Clinical insight

Patients can often find it difficult to localise abdominal pain. Ask them to use one finger to point to the area of maximum pain.

Pain	Location	Character or description
Appendicitis	Initially periumbilical, migrating to the right iliac fossa	Constant Associated with anorexia
Abdominal aortic aneurysm	May present as abdominal or back pain	Severe, sudden onset pain
Biliary colic	Right upper quadrant or epigastric	Severe and colicky Worse after eating fatty foods
Bladder	Suprapubic	Diffuse and severe
Bowel ischaemia	Right upper quadrant or central	Dull, severe and constant Exacerbated by eating
Colonic	Central	Colicky, associated with vomiting
Ectopic pregnancy	Right or left iliac fossa	Positive pregnancy test May be associated with vaginal bleeding
Intestinal obstruction	Central	Colicky, associated with vomiting and/or abdominal distension
Pancreatic	Epigastric, radiating to the back	Constant Often preceded by alcohol consumption
Peptic ulcer disease	Epigastric	Dull or burning pain Wakes the patient from sleep Exacerbated by eating
Peritonitic	Generalised, throughout abdomen	Patient lies still Keeps knees bent
Prostatic	Lower abdomen, rectum or perineum	Dull ache
Renal colic	Renal angles and/or loins, radiating to groins, testicles or labia	Severe pain Patient unable to keep still Paroxysms lasting 20–60 min

Table 5.2 Characteristic abdominal pains

(e.g. progressive or intermittent?). Ask the patient if the problem is found with solids or liquids.

Nausea and vomiting

Nausea is the unpleasant sensation of wanting to vomit. **Vomiting** is the forceful expulsion of the gastric contents caused by contractions of the thoracic and abdominal muscles. **Retching** differs from vomiting in that the contractions are present without expulsion of gastric contents. Identify the frequency and timing of nausea and vomiting. Is it acute or chronic? If vomiting is present, describe the quantity, colour and contents. **Haematemesis** is the vomiting of blood. Fresh blood is usually oesophageal; coffee-ground appearance suggests stomach or duodenal bleeding. Bilious vomit is green coloured and suggests obstruction. Bile is yellow as it leaves the ampulla of Vater. It then turns green in the stomach.

Diarrhoea and constipation

Identify the frequency, consistency and colour of the stool, and establish whether there has been any change. Stools can be described using the Bristol Stool Chart. Normal frequency of stools can be anything between three stools per day to three stools per week. **Diarrhoea** is an increase in stool volume (>200 mL/day) or frequency (more than two to three times a day). **Constipation** is a subjective complaint but can be defined as reduced frequency of defecation (less than three times a week) or the passage of stools that are hard and/or difficult to pass.

Rectal bleeding

Is the blood bright red (distal bleed or very large proximal bleed) or dark/black (also known as **melaena**, which signifies a proximal bleed)? Is the blood mixed with stool (e.g. colitis) or separate from stool (e.g. localised bleed)? Does the blood appear on the toilet paper (e.g. haemorrhoids) or in the toilet (e.g. cancer)?

Weight loss

Determine the following:
- Was the weight loss intentional?

- How much weight has been lost? (This may be reported in dropped clothes size)
- Diet: any changes, any exclusions, general content?
- Any associated symptoms?
- Stool changes?
- Signs of thyroid disease?

Signs

The key signs to elicit are demonstrated in **Table 5.3**.

General	Dehydration Pain	Cachexia or obesity Colour change
Hands	Clubbing Koilonychia Leukonychia Palmar erythema	Dupuytren's contracture Asterixis
Face	Oedema	Flushing
Eyes	Jaundice Anaemia	Kayser–Fleisher rings Xanthelasma
Mouth	Angular stomatitis Glossitis Poor dentition Ulcers	Sweet or foul-smelling breath Candidiasis
Neck	Lymphadenopathy	
Chest	Gynaecomastia	Spider naevi
Abdomen	Scars Masses Pain	Ascites Organomegaly Peristalsis or pulsations
Genitalia and groin	Hernias	Testicular mass, pain or swelling
Peripheries	Oedema Pyoderma gangrenosum	Erythema nodosum
Skin	Scratch marks	Bruising
Finish examination	Rectal examination	

Table 5.3 Key signs on abdominal examination

Jaundice

Jaundice is yellow discoloration that is best seen in the periphery of the ocular conjunctivae (sclera) or the oral mucosa. It is caused by excessive bilirubin in the circulation (**hyperbilirubinaemia**). It is often the first and only sign of liver disease and is therefore an important

> ## Clinical insight
>
> The cause of abdominal distension can be remembered using 6 Fs:
>
> F = fat (obesity)
>
> F = faeces (constipation)
>
> F = fetus (pregnancy)
>
> F = flatus (gas)
>
> F = fluid (ascites)
>
> F = freaky big tumour

clinical sign. Take a thorough history to identify the following:

- Is the jaundice associated with abdominal pain?
- Are there symptoms of biliary obstruction (pale stool and dark urine)?
- Have they had recent gastroenteritis (e.g. hepatitis A)?
- Any recent travel/unwell contacts?

The causes of jaundice can be split into pre-hepatic (e.g. Gilbert's syndrome), hepatocellular (e.g. cirrhosis) and post-hepatic causes (e.g. gallstones).

Gynaecomastia

Gynaecomastia is a benign proliferation of glandular breast tissue in men and must be differentiated from **pseudo-gynaecomastia**, which is excess fat deposition associated with obesity. Ask the patient to place his hands behind his head and palpate the nipple. In gynaecomastia a rubbery/firm mass will be palpable behind and extending from the nipple. It is associated with adolescence, drugs, cirrhosis and hypogonadism.

Abdominal distension

Abdominal distension is the generalised swelling of the abdomen. Note if the umbilicus is everted.

Ascites

Ascites is the accumulation of fluid in the peritoneal cavity. It is a common complication of liver cirrhosis. It is graded as follows:

- **Grade I:** mild ascites detectable only by ultrasound examination
- **Grade II:** moderate symmetrical distension of abdomen (shifting dullness present)
- **Grade III:** large or gross ascites with marked abdominal distension (fluid thrill present)

An ascitic tap (paracentesis) is often performed to identify the protein content (serum–ascites albumin gradient) and presence of blood.

5.3 Examination of the gastrointestinal system

Inspection

Positioning and exposure

- Ensure the patient is comfortable in the supine position with the arms resting by the patient's side
- The head should be comfortable and not flexed
- If necessary, place a pillow below bent knees to help the patient relax the abdominal muscles
- Expose the patient from the xiphisternum to the symphysis pubis
- Examine the genitalia independently once the abdomen has been examined

Classically, for abdominal examination, it has been said that the clinician should expose the patient 'from nipple to knees'. This can be embarrassing for the patient and a sheet should be placed over the genitals while examining the abdomen.

General inspection

Make an assessment of the patient's nutrition, looking particularly for signs of undernutrition (such as cachexia and muscle wasting) or obesity and then calculate the body mass index (BMI) (Chapter 2).

Eyes

Inspect the sclera for jaundice and the conjunctivae for pallor. Look for **Kayser–Fleischer rings** (greenish-yellow pigmentation encircling the corneoscleral junction, found in Wilson's disease due to copper deposition) and **xanthelasma** (raised yellow lesions caused by lipid deposition, seen around the eyes).

Hand and upper limb

Look particularly for Dupuytren's contracture, palmar erythema, nail signs (Table 2.8) and the presence of asterixis (Chapter 1). Examine the arms for signs of the following:

- **Spider naevi**: vascular lesions that comprise a central arteriole with surrounding smaller vessels, giving the appearance of a spider. They are classically found in the distribution of the superior vena cava (SVC), i.e. the trunk, face and upper limbs
- **Scratch marks**: these may suggest **pruritus** (excessive itchiness), often caused by cholestatic liver disease
- **Bruising**: this may be due to coagulation disorders resulting from hepatocellular damage or thrombocytopenia (found in hypersplenism)

The mouth

This is the only visible part of the alimentary canal. Inspect for dental disease, ulcers, sores and/or obvious candidal infection. Smell the patient's breath:

- **Ketosis**: sweet breath associated with high blood ketone levels
- **Uraemic fetor**: urine-like breath associated with high blood urea (**uraemia**)
- **Fetor hepaticus**: a sweet, faecal smell associated with liver disease

The abdomen

Inspect the abdomen for obvious distension, masses, pulsations, distended veins, stomas or scars (**Figure 5.3**). There should be a natural rise and fall of the abdomen during inspiration and expiration. A still abdomen may suggest peritonitis. Obvious, visible, peristaltic movements may suggest intestinal obstruction. Ask the patient to cough while observing the face for signs of pain and observing the abdomen for any changes in appearance (e.g. accentuation of masses). Similarly, ask the patient to lift the head off the bed (in order to increase abdominal pressure) and look for any obvious abdominal masses or hernias.

If there are prominent veins over the abdomen, note their location and determine the direction of blood flow. Inferior flow suggests SVC obstruction, superior flow suggests inferior

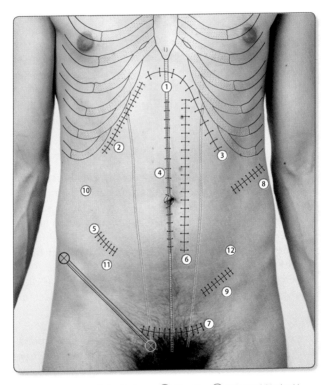

Figure 5.3 Common abdominal scars: (**1**), Line alba; (**2**), subcostal (Kocher's) incision; (**3**), extension of subcostal incision (double Kocher/roof top); (**4**), vertical midline incision; (**5**), transverse skin crease incision at McBurney's point; (**6**), paramedian incision; (**7**), suprapubic (Pfannenstiel's) incision; (**8**), renal; (**9**), left inguinal; (**10**), nephrostomy position; (**11**), ileostomy/urostomy position; (**12**), colostomy position; ⊗, anterosuperior iliac spine; ⊗, pubic tubercle.

vena cava (IVC) obstruction and **caput medusae** (flow radiating from the umbilicus) suggests portal vein hypertension.

The groin

Inspect the hernial orifices and genitalia for any abnormalities (Chapter 6).

Auscultation

Auscultation during the abdominal examination does not have the same level of importance as in a respiratory or cardiovascular examination. It is appropriate to auscultate before palpation because it has been argued that palpation of the abdomen may disturb intestinal peristalsis and therefore alter the bowel sounds.

Bowel sounds

The stethoscope can be placed on one site of the abdominal wall because there is no compartmentalisation of bowel sounds. Some clinicians choose to listen in all four quadrants. Normal peristaltic bowel activity produces characteristic 'gurgling' sounds (**borborygmi**) which can be heard every 2–10 seconds. Auscultate for bowel sounds for a minimum of 1 min before describing them as absent. Assess the following:

- Are the bowel sounds present or absent? Absence suggests an **ileus** (loss of normal peristaltic activity of the GIT). Paralytic ileus may be caused by peritonitis
- Quality of sounds: high-pitched or tinkling sounds can suggest bowel obstruction

Bruits

Bruits are heard over areas of turbulent blood flow within a vessel. They may be pathological, especially in the presence of hypertension. They can be heard just above and 2 cm lateral to the umbilicus on either side (**renal artery stenosis**) or just above the umbilicus (**abdominal aortic aneurysm**).

Palpation

Before palpating the abdomen, ask if the patient has any abdominal pain. Using warm hands, perform superficial palpation

(**Figure 5.4a**) in each of the four quadrants (**Figure 5.1b**), followed by deep palpation (**Figure 5.4b**). Superficial palpation will usually identify pain and/or guarding, and deep palpation masses and/or structural abnormalities. If a mass is palpable, describe it (Table 2.7). Ensure that the mass is not an enlarged organ.

Pain

Palpate the painful area last. Always observe the patient's face while palpating the abdomen, because this will reveal areas of

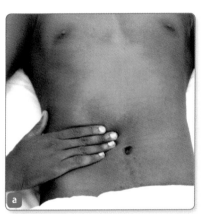

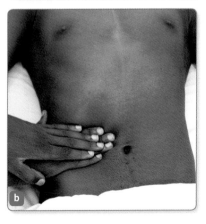

Figure 5.4 Abdominal palpation: (a) superficial palpation: eliciting any superficial tenderness. Palpate all four quadrants. (b) Deep palpation: eliciting deep tenderness, masses or organs. Palpate all four quadrants.

subtle tenderness. If the patient is guarding voluntarily, distract him or her with conversation. If pain is present, then assess for pathological signs (**Table 5.4**).

Liver

Place a flat hand at the most inferolateral position of the right lower quadrant (**Figure 5.5a**). Palpate gently and hold the hand in this position. Ask the patient to take a deep breath. The liver and spleen both move downwards on inspiration and would be felt to descend onto the index finger of the palpating hand. To correctly identify the liver, continue to palpate upwards in steps of 1–2 cm towards the costal margin, asking the patient to breathe in with each movement. Enlargement of the liver, **hepatomegaly**, is normally described in number of centimetres below the costal margin (**Table 5.5**).

To palpate the gallbladder, place your fingertips under the costal margin in the midclavicular line. Ask the patient to take a large inspiratory breath. A normal gallbladder is not palpable.

Term	Explanation	Implication
Abdominal guarding	Abdominal palpation leads to involuntary reflex contraction of the muscles of the abdominal wall	Peritonitis
Rebound tenderness (Blumberg's sign)	Slowly palpate into the abdomen Releasing the hand causes sudden acute pain Abdominal pain on coughing (cough sign) is a similar sign	Peritonitis
Rovsing's sign	Palpation of the left lower quadrant increases pain in the right lower quadrant	Appendicitis
McBurney's point tenderness	McBurney's point is found a third of the way from the right superior iliac spine to the umbilicus	Appendicitis
Murphy's sign	Pain in the midclavicular line at the right costal margin which is exacerbated by (or limits) deep inspiration	Cholecystitis

Table 5.4 Terminology related to abdominal pain

	Kidney	Spleen	Liver
Direction of enlargement	To flanks	To right iliac fossa	To right iliac fossa
Movement	Descends inferiorly on late inspiration	Descends inferomedially on early inspiration	Descends on early inspiration
Can you palpate above it?	Yes	No	No
Percussion	Resonant (bowel lying over it)	Dull	Dull
Pulsatile	No	No	Potentially
Expansile	No	No	Potentially
Additional features	Ballotable	Notch	None

Table 5.5 Differentiation of organomegaly

Spleen

The thoracic cage protects the spleen and it is therefore not normally palpable in the abdomen. If the tip is palpable, then the spleen is already enlarged two to three times its normal size. The spleen enlarges in the direction of the **right iliac fossa** (RIF). Therefore, to palpate the spleen, start in the RIF and continue upwards in the direction of the supralateral aspect of the left upper quadrant (**Figure 5.5a**). Use a similar technique to liver palpation, asking the patient to breathe in, keeping your hand still and allowing the spleen to descend onto your hand. The spleen should be differentiated from a palpable kidney (**Table 5.5**). If the spleen is palpable then **splenomegaly** is present and this should be classified.

Classification of splenomegaly

- **Grade I** (tip enlargement): spleen is palpable under the costal margin
- **Grade II** (moderate enlargement): spleen is palpable between the costal margin and the umbilicus
- **Grade III** (marked enlargement): spleen is palpable below the umbilicus

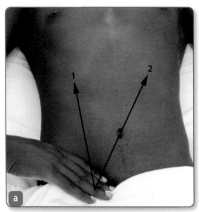

Figure 5.5 Palpation for organomegaly: (a) (1) liver palpation: start at right lower quadrant (RLQ) and palpate superiorly to the right upper quadrant (RUQ). (2) Spleen palpation: start at RLQ and palpate superiorly to the left upper quadrant (LUQ). (c) Right kidney (bimanual palpation): left hand placed under the patient's back and pushes up while the right hand rests on the patient's abdomen (opposite hands for left kidney).

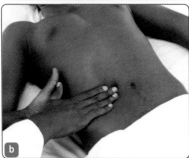

Kidneys

Use bimanual palpation to palpate the kidneys (**Figure 5.5b**). With the hands held in this position bring the two hands together (**ballot**). If a left-sided kidney is palpable, it should be differentiated from the spleen (**Table 5.5**).

Urinary bladder

It is not normal to palpate the bladder. In urinary retention, the bladder can be palpated rising out of the pelvis in the midline. It is not possible to get below the bladder. It is dull to percussion because it is fluid filled. A distended bladder is identified by a combination of palpation and percussion. In women of reproductive age it is worth considering the enlarged uterus of pregnancy.

Abdominal aorta

With the patient supine, use one hand to palpate between the umbilicus and xiphoid for an obvious **abdominal aortic aneurysm** (AAA). If a pulsing structure is palpable, then the size and direction of pulsation should be approximated. Place one hand on either side of the pulsatile structure (**Figure 5.6**). The fingers move outwards with a pulsatile mass (e.g. aorta) and upwards if the pulsation is transmitted through other tissues. Abdominal palpation for an aortic aneurysm is not accurate for dilatation <5 cm. Accuracy is further reduced in patients of larger body habitus.

Percussion

Percussion is performed using the same technique described in Chapter 1 (page 35). The percussion sounds will be dull for solid structures (e.g. liver) and fluids (e.g. ascites), or tympanitic (drum like) over air-filled structures (e.g. bowels). Also note if percussion causes pain because this would support other features of inflammation (e.g. peritonitis). Determining accurate percussion sounds will be difficult in obesity where subcutaneous fat impedes the transmission of the percussion note.

Liver and spleen

Percussion is used to determine the size of the liver and spleen and any abnormal gas collections. For liver size, percuss inferiorly from the breast in the midclavicular line (**Figure 5.7**).

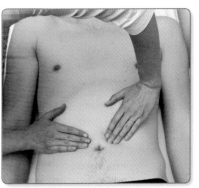

Figure 5.6 Palpation for abdominal aorta.

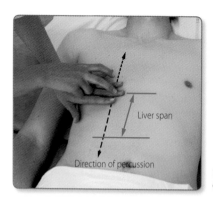

Figure 5.7 Percussion for organomegaly.

Once the superior edge has been identified, palpate for the inferior border of the liver and confirm this with percussion. A normal liver size is 10–12 cm in an adult. A similar method can be used to percuss the spleen at the left costal margin.

Shifting dullness

Shifting dullness is performed to identify ascites (**Figure 5.8**). It works on the principle that the gas-filled gut floats upwards with the free peritoneal fluid accumulating downwards:

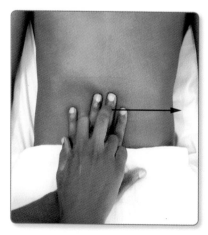

Figure 5.8 Eliciting shifting dullness.

1. Position the patient in the supine position
2. Percuss away from yourself, from umbilicus out towards the flank
3. When dullness is first detected, keep your fingers in that position and ask the patient to roll towards you
4. Wait a few seconds
5. If ascites is present, the dull percussion note should have become resonant (i.e. it 'shifts')

Shifting dullness is not a sensitive test (i.e. not good for ruling out ascites). There needs to be approximately 2 L of ascitic fluid for shifting dullness to be present. However, it is a specific test (i.e. good for ruling in ascites).

Fluid thrill or wave

Ask the patient (or colleague) to place the ulnar border of the hand firmly in the midline of the patient's abdomen (**Figure 5.9**). This prevents the thrill being artificially transmitted through soft tissues. Flick or tap one side of the patient's abdomen while feeling on the other side of the abdomen for the transmitted thrill. A positive test suggests a large volume of ascites. Not all cases of ascites will manifest a fluid thrill.

Digital rectal examination

Obtain informed consent and ensure that a chaperone is present. Avoid deferring the examination because you or the

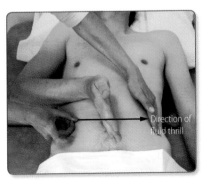

Direction of fluid thrill

Figure 5.9 Eliciting a fluid thrill.

patient finds it unpleasant. As it is an embarrassing and intimate examination, explain it to the patient before and during the procedure:

1. Give the patient some tissue, ready to wipe him- or herself afterwards
2. Position the patient in the left lateral decubitus position, with the hips and knees flexed and the gluteal muscles at the edge of the examining coach
3. Using a good light source, inspect the anal area for scars, fissures, fistulae, skins lesions, abscesses and/or haemorrhoids. Is there any obvious faecal soiling, mucus or blood present? If a fissure is present, then local anaesthetic gel should be applied before digital rectal examination
4. Ask the patient to 'Strain like you are passing a stool' and inspect for any obvious prolapse
5. Warn the patient and insert the tip of a lubricated, gloved, right index finger into the anal canal (**Figure 5.10a**)
6. Ask the patient to strain on the finger to assess sphincter tone and power; this is important for neurological examination
7. Warn the patient, and advance the finger fully into the rectum. Perform a 360° palpation of the anal and rectal walls (**Figure 5.10b**)
8. Describe any lesions noted (Table 2.7). Describe any lesion in terms of percentage of the rectal circumference involved and the distance of the diseased area from the anal canal
9. In men, palpate the anteriorly situated prostate, which is felt through the rectum. It should be smooth with a firm consistency. There is a shallow sulcus between the lateral lobes
10. After withdrawal, inspect your gloved finger for stool, blood and/or mucus

Clinical insight

There are three main abnormal findings on prostate examination:

1. **Benign prostatic hyperplasia**: smooth, enlarged prostate with intact sulcus
2. **Prostate cancer**: unilateral or bilateral irregular and/or nodular lobe(s) with possible loss of central sulcus
3. **Prostatitis**: enlarged, tender, boggy gland

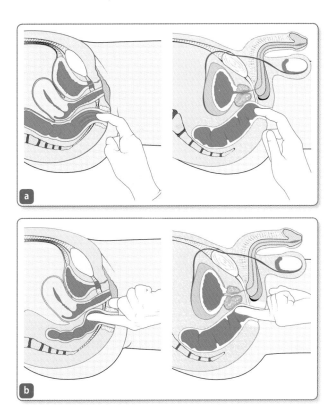

Figure 5.10 Digital rectal examination: (a) insertion of the finger (test for anal tone). (b) The hand is then rotated.

Proctoscopy

Proctoscopy is the visual inspection of the rectum and anal canal using a proctoscope. The mucosal lining of the normal rectum is similar to that of the buccal mucosa: red/pink, shiny and smooth. During retraction of the proctoscope, ask the patient to strain downwards to reveal haemorrhoids and/or rectal prolapse.

Prostate examination

As part of the male rectal examination, palpate the anteriorly situated prostate which is felt through the rectum. It should be smooth with a firm consistency. There is a shallow sulcus between the two lateral lobes.

5.4 Common investigations

Common investigations for gastrointestinal disease include:

- **Stool tests**: faecal occult blood (detects bleeding anywhere in the GIT and may indicate GI tract cancer), culture (for bacterial infection) and microscopy (for nematode parasites, Giardia, etc.)
- **Liver function tests**: plasma levels of proteins produced by the liver or associated with its damage (routinely including albumin, total protein, alanine transaminase, aspartate transaminase, alkaline phosphatase, bilirubins, gamma glutamyl transpeptidase and prothrombin time)
- **Pancreatic damage**: reflected by increased plasma concentrations of amylase
- **Amylase level**: raised in pancreatitis
- **Urine dipstick**: and microscopy, culture and sensitivity
- **Abdominal radiography**: to assess changes in bowel gas pattern and viscera, or to visualise conditions such as bowel perforation or obstruction (note the high radiation exposure, equivalent to 35 chest radiographs). Barium/contrast used for additional diagnostic information
- **Abdominal ultrasound**: to examine the viscera (Doppler ultrasound additionally visualises impaired blood flow, e.g. in renal artery stenosis)
- **Endoscopy**: to view the oesophagus, stomach and duodenum, for example in suspected cancer, dysphagia, acid reflux or upper GI bleed

> ## Clinical insight
>
> If perforation is suspected then an erect chest radiograph is the most sensitive study to detect free gas in the abdomen. If a patient is too sick to position erect, then a **decubitus** (on the side) image can be performed.

- **Colonoscopy**: to view the rectum, sigmoid and descending colon, for example identifying signs of ulceration, polyps and cancer
- **Endoscopic retrograde cholangiopancreatography**: to view the pancreatobiliary ducts, for example demonstrating obstruction due to gallstones or pancreatobiliary cancer
- **Renal function tests**: blood concentrations of urea and creatinine, along with electrolytes (sodium, potassium, chloride and bicarbonate). Glomerular filtration rate can be estimated from blood creatinine level

5.5 System summary

A summary of the abdominal examination is given in **Table 5.6**.

General	Wash hands; ensure privacy; introduce self and explain examination Gain consent for examination; offer a chaperone; position patient (supine with knees bent) and expose area being examined
Vital signs	Temperature; pulse rate; blood pressure; respiratory rate; oxygen saturation (what is their inspired oxygen?); capillary refill time (in children)
Inspection	Inspection of environment; general comfort; hands; face; mouth; neck (lymphadenopathy); abdomen; lower limbs
Auscultation	Bowel sounds; aortic and renal bruits
Palpation	Ask about pain (always watch patient's face while palpating abdomen) Light palpation; deep palpation; rebound tenderness; liver; spleen; ballot kidneys; bladder; abdominal aorta; lymph nodes (all regions).
Percussion	Shifting dullness; fluid thrill; liver; spleen; bladder
Complete the examination	Genitalia; hernial orifices; rectal examination including inspection of perianal region (do not assess in children as a student) Nutritional assessment; urinalysis Thank and cover the patient, and wash your hands

Table 5.6 Examination of the abdomen: a summary

Genitourinary system

The genitourinary (GU) system includes the organs of the urinary and reproductive systems. There is, therefore, overlap of the abdominal, GU and female reproductive examinations. This chapter focuses on the male aspects of the GU system.

6.1 System overview

Anatomy review

The urinary tract

The urinary tract comprises the kidneys, ureters, bladder and urethra. The urethra is shorter in women. This, combined with the urethral exit being closer to the anus (source of enteral bacteria), makes urinary tract infections (UTIs) more common in women.

The inguinal canal

The inguinal canal (**Figure 6.1**) is approximately 4 cm in length and allows the passage of the spermatic cord (three layers of fascia, ductus deferens, testicular artery, pampiniform plexus of veins, lymphatics and autonomic nerves) through the lower abdominal wall, obliquely through the deep inguinal ring, followed by the canal and then the superficial inguinal ring.

The prostate

The prostate is approximately the size of a walnut and surrounds the prostatic urethra (**Figure 5.10**). The prostate provides alkaline secretions to the seminal fluid. There are anterior, posterior, middle and lateral lobes of the prostate. On rectal examination the lateral lobes can be palpated, separated by a midline groove.

The testicle

The scrotal sac contains the terminal spermatic cords, testes and epididymis.

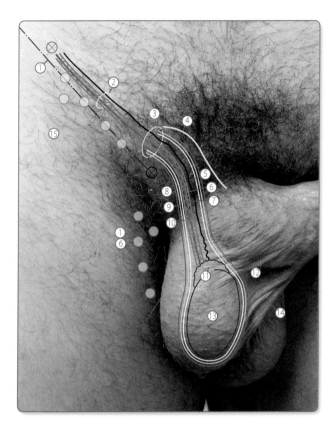

Figure 6.1 The inguinal canal: ①, inguinal ligament; ②, spermatic cord in the inguinal canal; ③, spermatic cord emerging from superficial inguinal ring; ④, ductus deferens; ⑤, pampiniform plexus; ⑥, testicular artery; ⑦, external spermatic fascia; ⑧, cremasteric fascia (external oblique); ⑨, cremasteric fascia (internal oblique); ⑩, internal spermatic fascia (transversalis fascia); ⑪, epididymis (head); ⑫, skin of scrotum; ⑬, testicle (surrounded by the tunica vaginalis); ⑭, midline scrotal raphe; ⑮, horizontal group of lymph nodes; ⑯, vertical group of lymph nodes; ⊗, position of deep inguinal ring; ⊗, pubic tubercle.

6.2 Symptoms and signs

Take a full history (**Table 6.1**) using the mnemonic OPERATES+ (Table 1.2) for each presenting complaint or problem.

Genitourinary symptoms

Pain on micturition

Dysuria is pain on **micturition** (passing urine). Identify where the pain is felt. Most often it is a burning pain at the urethral exit.

Haematuria

Haematuria is the passage of blood in the urine. It can be **macroscopic** (i.e. visible to the naked eye), or **microscopic** (i.e. found on urine dipstick testing or microscopy). It results from bleeding anywhere along the renal tract and should always be investigated.

Lower urinary tract symptoms

Frequency is the desire to pass urine more frequently than is normal for the patient. **Urgency** is the sudden, overwhelming desire to pass urine. **Nocturia** is urination during the night (quantify the frequency and volume of nocturnal urination).

As well as frequency, urgency and nocturia, an abnormal prostate may cause **hesitancy** (difficulty in starting the flow

History component	Key points
Presenting complaint	Urinary symptoms: dysuria, frequency, urgency, nocturia Haematuria Urinary incontinence Sexual function and/or libido Ease of passage of urine (prostatic features) Urethral discharge Testicular lump
Past medical history	Sexually transmitted infections Vascular, neurological and renal disease Menstrual history in women (page 143) Diabetes
Past surgical history	History of surgery
Social history	Current or previous tobacco use (quantify it in pack-years) Sexual history if appropriate (page 130) Occupational history (bladder cancer)

Table 6.1 The genitourinary history

of urine), poor stream, a disruption in flow or **terminal dribbling** (slow flow at the end of micturition). There may also be **incomplete bladder emptying** (the sensation of needing to void immediately after urinating). Identify whether the patient needs to strain or push when urinating.

Urethral discharge

Men may experience a urethral discharge. Enquire about the colour, consistency, smell and frequency of the discharge. Take a full sexual history (see below).

Sexual function

In practice, people have different understandings of problems with sexual function and the terminology can mean different things to different people. Enquire about sexual function in both males and females. If the patient is experiencing difficulty with sexual function enquire about the four stages of the sexual response cycle:

1. desire, arousal or excitement
2. plateau
3. orgasm
4. resolution

Dysfunction in these areas can be described as **loss of libido** (sexual desire), **erectile dysfunction** (the failure to establish or maintain an erection) or the inability to achieve orgasm.

Testicular pain

Use the SOCRATES mnemonic to take a pain history (Table 1.3). Is it associated with swelling, dysuria or haematuria? Testicular carcinoma and torsion must be ruled out.

The sexual history

This is a difficult history to take and requires patience and sensitivity. A sexual history is often required from both men and women to determine the risk of acquiring a **sexually transmitted infection** (STI) and/or pregnancy. The patient should be reassured about privacy and confidentiality.

Current sexual activity

The following questions should be asked about each sexual partner in the preceding 3 months (or most recent sexual partner if no sexual activity in previous 3 months):

- Gender of partner(s): don't make assumptions because of the gender of the patient
- Most recent sexual activity:
  - when (date)
  - penetrative or non-penetrative activity?
  - if penetrative: vaginal, anal and/or oral?
  - for each type of activity: was barrier contraception used?
  - other contraceptives used
- Nationality of partner?
- Does the patient or partner use illicit intravenous drugs?
- Does the partner have any symptoms or diagnosis?
- Has the partner had any other new partners?
- Has the patient or partner paid for or been paid for sex?

Past sexual history

- Age of first sexual activity
- Any sexual activity in a foreign country?
- Previous STIs
- Previous investigation for STIs (swabs and/or blood tests)
- Immunisations against hepatitis

Signs

The signs of GU disease are different in men (**Table 6.2**) and women (Chapter 7).

6.3 Examination of the genitalia

GU examination should be carried out as part of abdominal examination (Chapter 5). For examination of the female genitalia, see Chapter 7. This section focuses on examination of the prostate during rectal examination.

Sign	Differentiating features	Causes
Painful penis	Redness and swelling of glans with or without difficulty retracting foreskin	Balanitis
	Difficulty retracting foreskin with or without redness or swelling	Phimosis
Painful testicle	Swollen, warm testicle, which hangs higher in the scrotum	Orchitis Testicular torsion
	A lump is normally palpable	Testicular carcinoma
Genital ulcer	Painful	Herpes simplex
	Painless	Syphilis
Scrotal swelling	Feels like a 'bag of worms'	Varicocele
	Transilluminates Painful	Hydrocele Orchitis
Scrotal lump	Painless lump separate from testicle	Epididymal cyst
	Painful or painless lump arising from testicle	Testicular carcinoma
	Sudden onset severe pain	Testicular torsion
Groin lump	Absent cough impulse Rubbery in texture	Lymph node
	Positive cough impulse Lies inferior to pubic tubercle	Femoral hernia
	Positive cough impulse Lies over interior or exterior inguinal ring	Inguinal hernia
	Tender swelling inferior to inguinal ligament	Psoas abscess

Table 6.2 Common or important male genitourinary signs

Inspection

Obtain consent and ensure that a chaperone is present. Perform a general inspection including inspection for **gynaecomastia** (page 111). Inspect the visible external genital region for any ulcers, skin changes or swellings.

Penis

Inspect the penis. Ask the patient to retract the foreskin to inspect the glans and urethral meatus (in **phimosis** this is often not possible due to tightening of the foreskin). The meatus should be at the tip of the glans. **Epispadias** is a urethra exiting on the dorsal side of the glans. **Hypospadias** is a urethral exit on the ventral side of the penis; it can exit anywhere between the glans and the perineum. Inspect for discharge. Palpate the shaft of the penis for masses. A band of fibrosis along the shaft can cause curvature, which is exacerbated during an erection, making intercourse difficult or painful.

Scrotum

Examine the scrotum with the patient standing. The left testicle naturally lies lower than the right. If there is an obvious swelling, use a pen torch to transilluminate it. This should be done in a darkened room. A **hydrocele** (free fluid in tunica vaginalis) and **epididymal cyst** can usually be transilluminated, whereas testicular tissues cannot.

> ### Clinical insight
> Always examine the scrotum if a man has acute abdominal pain because scrotal pain can radiate to the abdomen. Delayed diagnosis of testicular torsion can result in the patient requiring an orchidectomy.

Palpation

Testes

Palpate each testicle (**Figure 6.2b**) individually, using the thumb and two fingers of the right hand and describe any lesions (Table 2.7). Always consider testicular carcinoma if palpation reveals a testicular lump. Palpate the epididymis (**Figure 6.2a**) and the spermatic cord for any discrete lesions. If there is a scrotal swelling palpate the lesion. If you cannot palpate above the lesion, it is abdominal in nature (i.e. a hernia). If it is a hernia, attempt to reduce it by palpating the contents back into the abdomen. A **varicocele** will feel like a 'bag of worms' and is normally painless. If only one testicle is palpable, carefully palpate high in the scrotum and the inguinal canal before describing it as non-descended.

Cremasteric reflex With the patient supine or standing, use a pointed instrument (e.g. swab) to stroke inferiorly along the

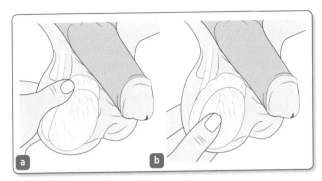

Figure 6.2 (a) Epididymis and (b) testicular palpation.

superomedial thigh, close to the testicles. A normal cremasteric reflex is an upward retraction of the ipsilateral testicle and scrotum. Upper and lower motor neurone disorders can cause an absence of the cremasteric reflex.

The inguinal region

The inguinal region should be inspected for obvious hernias. Ask the patient to cough and inspect for changes.

If there is an obvious herniation along the line of the spermatic cord or scrotum then:

- assess the consistency of the lump and any tenderness
- assess if coughing results in a palpable impulse
- ask the patient to reduce the hernia, if possible, by massaging it back through its source; the hernia should not reappear until pressure is released
- find and occlude the internal ring (**Figure 6.1**) and ask the patient to cough; if the lesion returns despite occlusion, then one can assume that this is a **direct inguinal hernia**

Femoral hernias are more common in women, and can easily strangulate. Examine them as for above (omitting the last step). If present, these hernias will appear as a lump lateral and inferior to the pubic tubercle. With the patient lying down, palpate for inguinal lymph nodes (see **Figure 6.1**).

6.4 Common investigations

Common investigations include:

- **Urine examination and dipstick** for signs of infection (e.g. white blood cells, red blood cells, protein)
- **Swabs** (urethral in men; urethral, vaginal, cervical and anal in women) to test for sexually transmitted infections, bacterial vaginosis and common infections
- **Blood tests for STIs**, for example HIV and syphilis
- **Prostate specific antigen and/or biopsy** for prostate irregularities
- **Ultrasound** for first-line visualisation of scrotal swellings, testicular lumps and femoral or inguinal hernias

6.5 System summary

A summary of the genitourinary examination is given in **Table 6.3**.

General	Wash hands; ensure privacy; introduce self and explain examination Gain consent for examination; offer a chaperone; position patient and expose area being examined
Inspection	Inspect penis (including retraction of foreskin to inspect the glans and meatus) Scrotum; inguinal region; inguinal canal and scrotum as patient coughs
Palpation	Testes; vas deferens; epididymis Cremasteric reflex; inguinal lympadenopathy Examine for hernias
Rectal examination	Position patient (left lateral position with knees drawn up) Inspect the perianal area and anus Assess sphincter tone; 180° 'sweep' in both directions Palpate the prostate in men (both lobes and the sulcus) Inspect glove after examination for evidence of blood, pus or mucus
Complete the examination	Urinalysis Thank and cover the patient and wash your hands

Table 6.3 Examination of the male genitalia and rectum: a summary

Female reproductive system

Although life expectancy is higher for women than men in most countries, a number of health and social factors combine to create a lower quality of life for women in many parts of the world. Breast cancer is the leading cause of cancer death among women aged 20–59 years in high-income countries. Examination of the female genital system involves unique skills that need to be practised in order to achieve competence. This chapter includes details on breast, gynaecological and obstetric history and examination.

Clinical insight

The patient may be embarrassed to talk about gender-specific health issues. Special care should be taken to make the patient feel comfortable and enable her to give a clear history. A chaperone (preferably female) should be present for any gynaecological examination. For breast, gynaecological and obstetric examination, start with general inspection, and respiratory and cardiovascular examinations. This is good practice and also allows time to develop a rapport and trust.

7.1 System overview

Anatomy review

Breast

The mammary gland (breast) is divided into four quadrants (**Figure 7.1**) by horizontal and vertical lines that intersect the nipple. A fifth area of tissue, the tail of Spence, extends laterally towards the axilla. The nipple is surrounded by the areola, a circular pigmented area. Milk-secreting glands within the breast tissue are drained by lactiferous ducts, which open onto the nipple.

Seventy-five per cent of lymphatic drainage of the breast, drains to the axillae. The remainder drains to the internal mammary nodes and the supraclavicular region.

Female genital system

The female pelvis (**Figure 7.2**) comprises the external genital organs (known as the vulva, vagina, uterus, fallopian tubes and

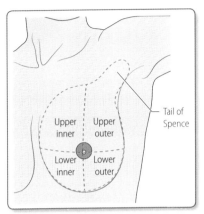

Figure 7.1 Quadrants of the breast.

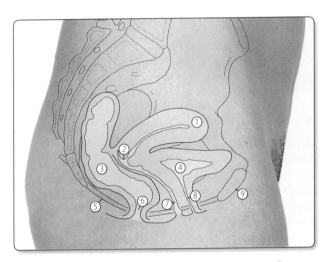

Figure 7.2 Organs of female pelvis: lateral view. (1), Fundus of uterus; (2), cervix of uterus; (3), rectum; (4), bladder; (5), levator ani (pelvic floor muscle); (6), anal canal (note change of angle at anorectal junction); (7), vaginal canal; (8), urethra; (9), pubic symphysis.

ovaries). The vagina lies posterior to the bladder and anterior to the rectum. The uterus comprises the cervix, body and fundus. It is most often found to be **anteverted** (the long axis of the uterus is angled forward), and in the nulliparous female it measures approximately $8 \times 5 \times 2.5$ cm. The fornices are the deepest part of the vagina and are found around the cervix. They are divided into anterior, posterior, and left and right lateral regions.

Physiology review
Normal breast changes
During puberty, oestrogen induces the development of the mammary ducts and distribution of the fatty tissue, whereas progesterone promotes alveolar growth. During pregnancy, oestrogen, progesterone and prolactin stimulate breast tissue growth. Prolactin promotes milk production in the postnatal period.

Menstrual cycle
The menstrual cycle can be divided into three phases (**Figure 7.3**):
1. The **menstrual phase** starts on day 1 if fertilisation has not occurred. Progesterone and oestrogen levels fall and the endometrium will start to degenerate
2. The **proliferative (follicular)** phase starts at the end of menses (on about day 4) and ends at ovulation (on about day 14). Follicle-stimulating hormone (FSH) stimulates ovarian follicles to mature, while the endometrium thickens
3. The **luteal (secretory)** phase begins and lasts until day 28. A surge in luteinising hormone (LH) triggers ovulation and progesterone stimulates endometrial glands

7.2 The breast consultation

Take a full history (**Table 7.1**) using the mnemonic OPERATES+ (Table 1.2) for each presenting complaint. Establish the following features in relation to each symptom:
- Is the patient pregnant or breastfeeding?

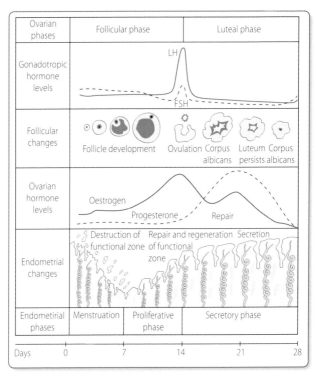

Figure 7.3 Menstrual cycle.

- Unilateral or bilateral?
- Relationship to menstrual cycle or is the patient postmenopausal?

Symptoms
Breast lump
Any breast lump must be thoroughly evaluated. This may consist of serial examinations in a younger patient but in an older woman, investigations should be promptly carried out. Establish when the lump was first noticed, any changes since then and

History component	Key points
Presenting complaint	Breast lump Breast pain Nipple discharge or bleeding Change in nipples (e.g. skin changes, in-drawing)
Past medical history	Breast disease Detailed menstrual history
Past surgical history	Previous breast surgery
Drug history	Hormonal contraceptive use Hormonal replacement therapy
Family history	Breast, ovarian or colon cancer
Social history	Current or previous tobacco use (quantify it in pack-years) Alcohol history

Table 7.1 The breast history

any associated symptoms. Causes of breast lump include the following:

- **Cyst:** smooth, spherical lump; can be painful
- **Fibroadenoma:** painless, smooth mass with rubbery consistency
- **Carcinoma:** painless, firm, irregular lump with skin tethering; skin changes or nipple discharge may be present
- **Fat necrosis:** firm, hard lump with skin tethering; occurs after trauma
- **Abscess:** painful, hot, red lump; often associated with breastfeeding

Clinical insight

Breast cancer is the most common cancer in women in both developed and resource-poor countries. Incidence increases with age. Consider that the presenting symptom may be one of metastasis (e.g. arm swelling due to lymphatic obstruction or cough due to lung infiltration).

Breast pain (mastalgia)

Take a pain history using the SOCRATES mnemonic (Table 1.3). Hormonal changes commonly cause pain in premenopausal women. Breast cancer is a rare but important cause of mastalgia.

Nipple discharge

Establish whether the discharge is milky in consistency (consistent with **galactorrhoea**). If a pituitary adenoma with galactorrhoea is suspected, ask about headaches and visual disturbance.

7.3 Examination of the breast

For breast and pelvic examinations, it is of particular importance to explain each step of the examination and continually check that the patient is comfortable before proceeding.

Inspection

Perform a general inspection of the patient (Chapter 2).

Inspection of the breast

Ask the patient to undress to the waist and sit on the edge of the examination table. Inspect the breasts with the patient in the following positions (**Figure 7.4**):

1. Sitting upright with the arms resting by her sides
2. Leaning forward, with her hands on her hips, first with hands relaxed then with her hands pressed into her hips ('pectoral contraction manoeuvre')

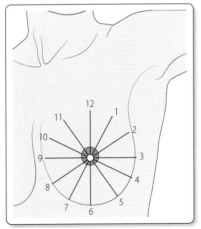

Figure 7.4 Breast inspection clock face for describing lesions.

3. With the hands behind her head (paying particular attention to the axilla)

Inspect for:

- size, symmetry and contour of breasts
- obvious lumps
- scars, discoloration, inflammation, displacement, prominent veins, puckering, dimpling or peau d'orange

Inspection of the nipples

Inspect for asymmetry, inversion, discharge or scale (this can indicate **Paget's disease** of the breast).

Palpation

Palpation of the breast

Palpate the asymptomatic breast first. Position the patient at 45° and place her hand behind her head on the side that you are examining (**Figure 7.4**). Palpate the breast using the flat of your three middle fingers. Be systematic and palpate all four breast quadrants, beneath the areola and finally the axillary tail. You can use either a concentric circular pattern or examine each half of the breast from the superior edge progressing downwards (**Figure 7.5**). Check the nipples for discharge. If you palpate a lump, describe its features using the SSS CCC FFF TTT mnemonic (Table 2.7). When noting the location of any lump, describe the location in terms of its position on a clock face, e.g. 'the lump is in the 4 o'clock position' (**Figure 7.4**).

> ### Clinical insight
>
> Skin changes resulting from a tumour can include tethering or peau d'orange (skin resembling an orange peel). This is caused by lymphoedema and can be a sign of breast carcinoma or a result of radiotherapy to the breast.

> ### Clinical insight
>
> Taking a good menstrual history is central to many of the health issues related to women's health:
>
> - Age of onset of menstruation (menarche)
> - Date of the first day of their last menstrual period (LMP)
> - Duration and frequency (e.g. 5 out of 28 days)
> - Flow – heavy or light (ask about clots, and use of both tampons and pads, which suggests heavy flow)
> - Irregular bleeding (e.g. intermenstrual or postcoital)
> - Menstrual pain (breast and/or pelvic)
> - Change in cycle since menarche
> - Age of menopause (if applicable)

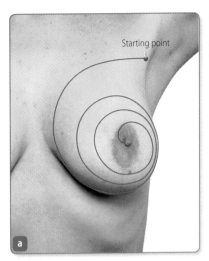

Figure 7.5 Breast palpation: systematic approach using (a) concentric circular path, starting in tail of Spence or (b) each half sequentially.

Starting point

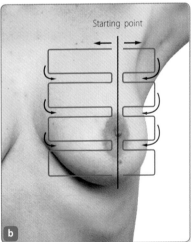

Starting point

Complete the examination

Inspect and palpate the axillae (**Figure 2.4c**) and supraclavicular (**Figure 2.4b**) regions for lymphadenopathy. If you feel a breast lump, then you should examine the spine, abdominal and neurological systems for evidence of metastatic spread.

7.4 The gynaecological consultation

Use the mnemonic OPERATES+ (Table 1.2) to gain a full presenting history and then take a full gynaecological history (**Table 7.2**). In addition, establish if there is any change in symptoms in relation to the menstrual cycle.

Symptoms
Abnormal bleeding

Ask about flow, associated pain (**dysmenorrhoea**) and timing of abnormal bleeding: is it **intermenstrual** (IMB) or **postcoital** (PCB). IMB and PCB may be symptoms of cervical cancer. Any patient with postmenopausal bleeding must be evaluated for uterine cancer. Establish whether **amenorrhoea** is primary or secondary.

Urinary incontinence

Urinary incontinence is commonly due to stress incontinence or detrusor overactivity. **Incontinence** is the involuntary voiding of urine. There are several types:

- **Overflow incontinence:** loss of urine from a chronically distended bladder
- **Stress incontinence:** increased abdominal pressure (e.g. from coughing), causing leakage of urine
- **Urge incontinence:** associated with urgency; patient unable to reach the toilet quickly enough
- **True incontinence:** a complete loss of control of the bladder

When taking a history it is important to differentiate between loss of control and the inability to reach or identify an appropriate facility.

Pelvic pain

Use the SOCRATES mnemonic (Table 2.3). Pain may be acute or chronic and is often associated with **dyspareunia** (painful intercourse). Dyspareunia may be superficial (pain on penetration) or deep (felt in the pelvis).

History component	Key points
Presenting complaint	Abnormal bleeding Menorrhagia Dysmenorrhoea Amenorrhoea Irregular bleeding Postmenopausal bleeding Postcoital bleeding Vaginal discharge Pelvic pain Dyspareunia Vulval symptoms, e.g. itch Genital prolapse Urinary symptoms: dysuria, frequency, urgency, incontinence Subfertility
Past gynaecological history	Cervical smears (any abnormal smears and date of last smear) Gynaecological problems (including any surgery) Sexually transmitted infections
Past obstetric history	Gravidity and parity Any problems in pregnancy or labour Outcome of all pregnancies
Past medical history	Anaemia Bowel complaints
Past surgical history	Abdominal surgery
Drug history	Hormone replacement therapy Contraception Alternative therapies or over-the-counter medications
Family history	Breast, colon or ovarian cancer, diabetes or hypertension
Social history	Current or previous tobacco use (quantify it in pack-years) Sexual history Domestic violence (women will often not disclose this voluntarily, so it must be asked about in a sensitive way when the woman is alone)

Table 7.2 The gynaecological history

Vaginal discharge

Ask about colour, odour, volume, presence of blood and any associated irritation.

Infective causes of discharge are as follows:

- **Bacterial vaginosis:** grey, watery and fishy smelling
- *Candida albicans:* thick, white and associated with vulval irritation
- *Trichomonas vaginalis:* yellow, frothy and fishy smelling
- **Chlamydia infection:** copious, purulent discharge (but asymptomatic in 80% of women)
- **Gonorrhoea:** purulent discharge (but asymptomatic in 50% of women)

7.5 The gynaecological examination

The gynaecological examination is made up of four sections: abdominal (Chapter 5), external genitalia, vaginal and speculum examination. The patient should void urine before a vaginal/pelvic examination. Ensure that there is good lighting. Position the women in the lithotomy position (**Figure 7.6**). Always wear gloves for these examinations.

Inspection (external genitalia)

Separate the labia majora to inspect the external genitalia (**Figure 7.7**). Also inspect the labia minora, introitus, urethral meatus and clitoris for:

- atrophy
- discharge or bleeding
- inflammation
- lumps or masses
- plaques
- scars
- trauma
- ulceration

Clinical insight

Lithotomy position: This position is used for pelvic examinations and many surgical procedures. The patient is supine with the perineum at the edge of the examination couch. The feet are positioned at, or slightly above, the level of the pelvis. In theatre, this is achieved with stirrups.

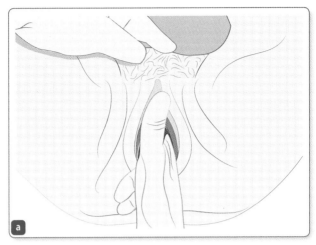

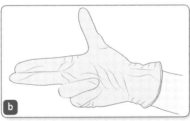

Figure 7.6 Bimanual palpation: (a) lithotomy position of patient, (b) hand position used for bimanual palpation.

Ask the patient to cough or strain down to evaluate for prolapse and/or incontinence.

Speculum examination

Cusco's (bivalve) speculum is a gynaecological instrument that is used to inspect the cervix and vagina. Clear plastic speculums are becoming more popular because they are single use, disposable and offer better views of the vaginal wall through the clear plastic.

Inspection

Gently part the labia with one hand and insert a warm lubricated speculum with your other hand. The blades should be

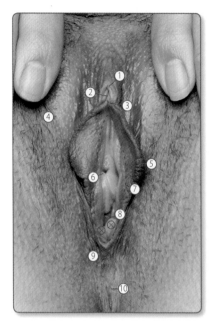

Figure 7.7 Female external genitalia, vaginal vestibule: ①, Prepuce of clitoris; ②, glans of clitoris; ③, frenulum of clitoris; ④, labia majora (opened); ⑤, labia minora; ⑥, external urethral orifice; ⑦, margin of vaginal vestibule (blue line); ⑧, vaginal orifice; ⑨, posterior commissure of labia/fourchette; ⑩, perineal body; X, opening of greater vestibular gland ducts.

closed and parallel with the vagina. Once inserted, rotate the speculum 90° so that the handle is pointing upwards. Gently open the blades and, once you have visualised the cervix, secure them in place. If you are unable to visualise the cervix, try asking the patient to cough. If still unable to visualise the cervix, perform a bimanual examination (see below) to locate the cervix and then repeat the speculum examination.

Inspect the cervix for:

- colour (should be pink)
- regularity
- os (open or closed)
- inflammation
- bleeding or discharge
- ulceration or erosions
- growths

Before removing the speculum it may be necessary to take tests for sexually transmitted infections (STIs) and/or perform a cervical (Pap) smear. Withdraw the speculum, while rotating it back 90°. Take note of the vaginal walls as you do so, looking for any obvious skin changes, abnormal growths or prolapse. As you remove the speculum, the blades should be allowed to close. Take care never to close the blades on the cervix, and not to pinch any skin or hair.

Smear and swabs

With the cervix visible do the following:

- Use a spatula and cytobrush to collect ectocervical and endocervical portions of the cervical smear
- Rotate the spatula or cytobrush 360° five times
- Remove the instruments while avoiding touching the speculum
- Drop the brush into the collection container

If STI testing is needed, collect an endocervical swab. A high vaginal swab may also be taken.

Palpation (vaginal and pelvic) examination

If there are any obvious masses, these will need to be palpated (Table 2.7).

Entering the vagina

Warn the patient that you are about to examine her internally and ask permission to continue:

- Gently separate the labia with the left hand
- Gently insert the index and middle finger of your gloved right hand into the vagina (**Figures 7.6** and **7.8**). Use lubricant. As you enter, your palm should be facing laterally; once fully inserted it can be rotated 90° to face upwards

Vagina and cervix

As you insert your fingers, palpate the vaginal walls for any irregularities or masses.

Find the cervix, which is usually pointing downwards in the upper vagina. It is said to resemble a 'nose', particularly in the nulliparous patient. Assess:

- consistency (hard or soft)
- os (open or closed)

- mobility
- position
- size
- cervical motion tenderness (CMT): this is pain on moving the cervix from side to side; this may be a sign of infection or ectopic pregnancy; anything that irritates the peritoneal lining can cause CMT (e.g. appendicitis)
- fornices – either side of the cervix

Bimanual examination

Place your left hand 4 cm above the symphysis pubis and push down. Position the fingers of the right hand in the posterior fornix and gently push upwards (**Figures 7.6** and **7.8**). Assess the uterus for:

- position (anteverted or retroverted)

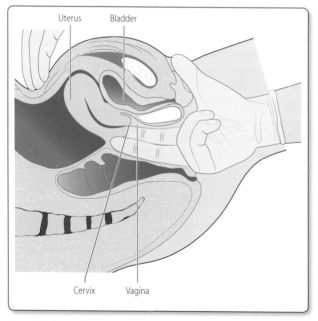

Figure 7.8 Bimanual palpation.

- size
- shape
- regularity
- tenderness

Palpate the adnexa (ovaries and fallopian tubes) bilaterally by placing the internal (right-hand) fingers in the fornix while placing the external (left) hand over the corresponding iliac fossa. The ovaries are often palpable on bimanual examination, but the fallopian tubes should not be palpable. If a mass is identified, assess for size, shape, mobility, masses and tenderness (adnexal tenderness may be a sign of infection). Finally, gently remove the fingers and inspect the glove for any blood or discharge.

7.6 The obstetric consultation

Take a full obstetric history (**Table 7.3**).

7.7 The obstetric examination

General examination

You should perform a general examination (Chapter 2), including cardiovascular and respiratory examination. Measure the blood pressure in the left lateral position at 45° to avoid compression of the inferior vena cava by the gravid uterus.

Clinical insight

When describing number of pregnancies ($G_n P_{TPAL}$):

G_n = total number of pregnancies

T = total number of term deliveries (≥37 weeks)

P = total number of preterm deliveries (20–37 weeks)

A = total number of abortions or miscarriages, including ectopic pregnancies (<20 weeks)

L = total number of living children

Inspection

Abdominal, vaginal and speculum examinations all make up important parts of the obstetric examination and are required at different points in pregnancy and labour. Use the aforementioned techniques of examination.

History component	Key points
Presenting complaint	Vaginal bleeding, discharge or leakage of fluid Abdominal pain or contractions Fetal movements (from 18 weeks to 20 weeks) Pre-eclampsia symptoms: headache, oedema, blurred vision, epigastric pain, vomiting or convulsions Minor symptoms of pregnancy, e.g. fatigue, nausea and vomiting, gastro-oesophageal reflux, constipation
Current pregnancy	How was pregnancy confirmed? First day of last menstrual period (LMP) Estimated due date (EDD): EDD = LMP + 9 months + 7 days Menstrual history Prior use of contraceptives Antenatal care: where, number of visits Dating and anomaly ultrasound scans Serological screening (HIV, hepatitis B, syphilis and rubella) Blood group or type, rhesus status and antibody screen
Past obstetric history	Gravidity and parity Any problems in pregnancy or labour Outcome of all pregnancies
Past medical history	Take a full medical history (Chapter 1), including medical, surgical and psychiatric problems Past gynaecological history (**Table 7.2**)
Past surgical history	Previous blood transfusions
Drug history	Immunisation history Drugs taken in pregnancy (prescribed or over the counter)
Family history	Congenital anomalies, diabetes, hereditary disorders
Social history	During pregnancy: smoking (in pack-years), alcohol consumption (how much and when) and illicit drug use Housing, financial situation and marital status Partner: name, age, occupation, medical problems Was the pregnancy planned? Has the woman presented late in her pregnancy?

Table 7.3 The obstetric history

Abdominal inspection

Assess:

- symmetry
- fetal movements
- scars – check carefully for Pfannenstiel's ('bikini-line') scar from previous caesarean section
- skin changes of pregnancy:
  - linea nigra: hyperpigmented line extending from pubic symphysis upwards in the midline
  - stretch marks: also known as striae gravidarum
- umbilical flattening and/or eversion

Palpation

Abdominal palpation

Ensure that there is no tenderness at the fundus (top) of the uterus.

Symphyseal–fundal height (uterine size) To identify the **fundus** move inferiorly from the sternum using the ulnar border of the left hand. Locate the upper border of the pubic symphysis with the right hand and measure between the two with a tape measure (**Figure 7.9**). This is expressed in centimetres as the **symphyseal–fundal height** and correlates to the number of weeks gestation between 16 and 36 weeks ($\pm$ 2 cm).

Fetal lie Face the mother's feet. Using both hands palpate, in steps, inferiorly down the uterus (**Figure 7.10a**). It takes practice to be able to find the smooth firm resistance of the back of the fetus versus the irregular shape of the limbs (**Figure 7.10b**). The head is palpable as a smooth round object that is ballotable between the hands. **Fetal lie** is the relationship between the long axis of the fetus and the uterus, and can be described as longitudinal (parallel to long axis of uterus), transverse (right angle to long axis of uterus) or oblique (45° to long axis of uterus).

Fetal presentation Still facing the patient's feet, palpate either side of the lower uterus to determine the presenting part (**Figure 7.10c**). It can be cephalic (vertex, brow or face), breech (bottom), shoulder, compound (more than one fetal part presenting, e.g. hand over head) or cord (funic) presentation.

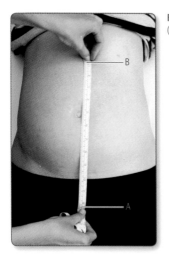

Figure 7.9 Symphyseal–fundal height: (a) pubic symphysis, (b) fundus.

Engagement This is usually assessed using Pawlick's grip (**Figure 7.10d**). You should stop if this causes pain. Engagement is the level of the fetal head in the pelvis and is usually described as 'fifths palpable'. One-fifth of a fetal head is equivalent to approximately one finger-breadth. If the entire head is palpable in the abdomen it is five-fifths palpable (i.e. not engaged). If none of the head is palpable in the abdomen, it is zero-fifths palpable (i.e. fully engaged). The fetal head typically engages days to weeks before labour in nulliparous patients.

Estimation of amniotic fluid volume Palpation of fetal parts will give an approximate indication of amniotic fluid volume. In **polyhydramnios** (increased fluid volume), the uterus is large compared with gestation and so fetal parts are less easily felt. In **oligohydramnios** (reduced fluid volume) the opposite is true.

Vaginal examination

Vaginal examination in labour is key to assessing cervical status and presentation of the fetus. By using the techniques described above, assess cervical:
- dilatation (up to 10 cm)

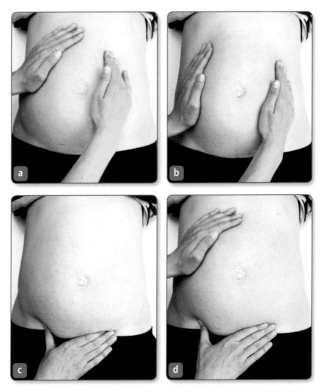

Figure 7.10 Obstetric palpation: (a) fetal lie, (b) fetal spine and extremities, (c) fetal presentation, (d) engagement and confirm fetal lie.

- length and effacement
- consistency

Finally, assess the station of the head in relation to the ischial spines (in centimetres). It may be above or below the spines.

Speculum examination

Speculum examination is used as required in pregnancy, e.g. in suspected labour to assess for rupture of membranes or during pregnancy to take swabs (if infection is suspected).

Auscultation

Fetal heart sounds are first heard at 11–12 weeks by a pocket Doppler and 16–19 weeks with a Deelee fetal stethoscope. The fetal heart rate (FHR) is normally 110–150 beats/min (bpm) and should be regular.

7.8 Common investigations

Common investigations include:

- **Pregnancy test**: performed on blood or urine by testing for β-human chorionic gonadotrophin
- **Urine dipstick (Table 5.6) and microscopy, culture and sensitivity**: to identify protein (pre-eclampsia), glucose (diabetes) and infection
- **Urine assays, blood serology and vaginal swabs**: to identify STIs
- **Glucose tolerance test:** if gestational diabetes is suspected
- **Cervical screening**: to identify premalignant conditions of the cervix
- **Colposcopy:** for direct and magnified inspection of the surface of the cervix, usually carried out by a specialist. Cervical biopsy can also be performed

7.9 System summary

A summary of all the female examinations is given in **Table 7.4**.

General	General	Wash hands; ensure privacy; introduce self and explain examination Gain consent for examination; ensure that a chaperone is present Position patient (supine) and expose area being examined
	Vital signs	Temperature; pulse rate; blood pressure; respiratory rate and oxygen saturation
	General inspection	Inspection of patient's environment; general comfort
Breast	Inspection	Inspection of breasts with patient sitting upright, hands on hips and then with arms behind head Nipples; axillae
	Palpation	Asymptomatic breast and axillary tail; symptomatic breast and axillary tail Axillary lymph nodes; cervical and supraclavicular lymph nodes
Gynaecological	Inspection	Abdominal inspection External genitalia Speculum examination
	Palpation	Palpation of abdomen
	Vaginal examination	Palpate and the vagina and cervix Bimanual examination
Obstetric	Inspection	Abdominal inspection (scars, symmetry, fetal movements, skin changes, umbilicus)
	Palpation	Symphyseal–fundal height; fetal lie; fetal presentation; engagement Estimation of amniotic fluid volume Vaginal examination (if appropriate); speculum examination (if appropriate)
	Auscultation	Doppler or Deelee/Pinard's stethoscope
	Complete the examination	General examination (cardiovascular, etc) Assessment of nutritional state; urinalysis Thank and cover the patient, and wash your hands

Table 7.4 Comprehensive female examination: a summary

Neurological system

The nervous system is one of the most complex systems of the body. It is responsible for our movements (voluntary and involuntary), hormonal regulation, senses, consciousness, reasoning and personalities. It is also one of the most difficult examinations to perform and therefore needs considerable practice.

8.1 System overview

Anatomy review

Central nervous system

Cortex The **cerebral cortex** is the grey matter that covers the hemispheres. The primary cortices (**Figure 8.1**) directly receive sensory information or are directly involved in movement initiation. The brain receives its blood supply from the carotid and vertebral arteries, which in turn supply the cerebral cortices via the cerebral arteries of the circle of Willis (**Figure 8.2**).

Motor pathways The direct (pyramidal) pathways are responsible for our voluntary movements. The upper motor neurone (UMN) originates in the cerebral cortex, descends through the

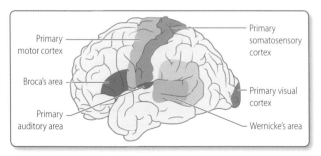

Primary motor cortex

Broca's area

Primary auditory area

Primary somatosensory cortex

Primary visual cortex

Wernicke's area

Figure 8.1 Major functioning areas of hemisphere.

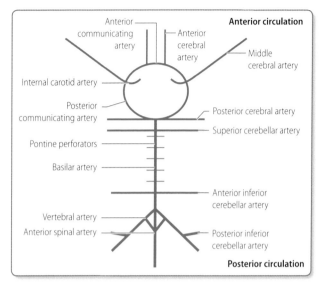

Figure 8.2 The circle of Willis.

internal capsule, brain stem and spinal cord, before synapsing with the lower motor neurone (LMN), which is responsible for innervating skeletal muscle.

The indirect (extrapyramidal) pathways involve a series of complex circuits of the central nervous system (CNS). These control movements in response to balance, muscle tone and visual stimuli.

Sensory pathways The **posterior columns** carry proprioception and vibration sense up the ipsilateral side of the spinal cord, along with some of the fibres responsible for light touch. The **lateral (spinothalamic) columns** decusatte (crossover) at the level of the pyramids and, therefore, carry pain and temperature sensation up the contralateral side of the spinal cord. A spinal nerve then arises at each spinal level, containing both sensory and motor neurones. An area of skin supplied by a single spinal level is known as a **dermatome** (**Figure 8.3**).

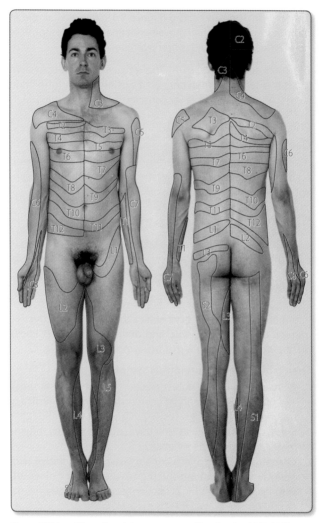

Figure 8.3 An evidence-based dermatome map. (Based on Lee MWL, McPhee RW, Stringer MD. An evidence-based approach to human dermatomes. Clin Anat 2008;21:363–73.)

Cerebellum The cerebellum (**Figure 8.1**) plays a vital role in motor control rather than movement initiation. It is responsible for balance, posture and motor learning.

Reticular activating system The reticular activating system (RAS) is a series of interconnected nuclei found in the brain stem that are responsible for consciousness.

Physiology review
Deep tendon reflexes
A reflex is a rapid, involuntary response to a stimulus. The deep tendon reflexes (also known as stretch reflexes) are monosynaptic reflexes that function at a spinal level.

8.2 Symptoms and signs

Take a full neurological history (**Table 8.1**) using the mnemonic OPERATES+ (Table 1.2) for each presenting complaint/problem.

Symptoms
The neurological examination can provide a great deal of information, but the history remains the single most effective method to localise a lesion(s) and/or make a diagnosis. Focus on the progress and timing of the symptoms.

Timing of onset of neurological symptoms
- **Acute** (seconds to minutes): electrical activity (e.g. seizures), vascular (e.g. subarachnoid haemorrhage), mechanical (e.g. trauma)
- **Subacute** (hours to days): infective (e.g. meningitis), inflammatory (e.g. multiple sclerosis)
- **Chronic** (months to years): neoplastic, degenerative (e.g. genetic disorders), endocrine (e.g. Cushing's disease), chronic infection or inflammation (e.g. tuberculosis)

Headache
This is the most common neurological symptom. Take a pain history using the SOCRATES mnemonic (Table 1.3). Enquire about visual symptoms, facial symptoms, weakness

History component	Key points
Presenting complaint	Headaches Fits, faints or funny turns Weakness (or unsteadiness) Dizziness and loss of balance Sensory symptoms (vision, hearing or taste) Transient loss of function (e.g. vision, speech or sight) Memory problems Paraesthesia Wasting of muscles Spasms Involuntary movements (e.g. tremors) Loss of sphincter control (urinary or bowel)
Past medical history	Epilepsy Psychiatric disease Cardiovascular disease
Past surgical history	History of cancer
Drug history	Antiepileptic medications, anti-dopaminergics, oral contraceptives, steroids, anticoagulants and psychiatric medications
Family history	Epilepsy Neurological disease Dementia
Social history	Current or previous tobacco use (Chapter 1) Current or previous illicit drug or alcohol abuse or addiction Driving status (this may need to be discussed after a diagnosis has been made)

Table 8.1 The neurological history

and/or numbness. A thorough social history is paramount to identify stressors or triggers. Timing can be useful to identify causes:

- single acute episode (e.g. bacterial or viral meningitis)
- repeated acute episodes (e.g. migraine)
- subacute (e.g. raised intracranial pressure)
- chronic (e.g. depression)

Fits, faints and funny turns

Seizures (fits), **syncope** (faints) and dizziness (funny turns) are common presenting complaints. Syncope is discussed in Chapter 3 (page 63). These episodes can be **epileptiform** in nature (e.g. generalised tonic–clonic seizure) or **non-epileptiform** (e.g. vasovagal). A third party history (e.g. from a bystander) is crucial because usually the patient has no, or only partial, recollection of the events.

A seizure history can be very difficult and is often done badly. Using the OPERATES+ mnemonic (Table 1.2) to take a history would be useful, but will not always identify all the pertinent information required. The history should be split into three time periods: pre-seizure, seizure and post-seizure.

Pre-seizure
- Any warning signs, e.g. visual disturbance?
- Was the onset sudden or gradual?
- What was the patient doing at the time, e.g. had they just stood from sitting?
- What was their posture immediately before, i.e. sitting or standing?
- Had the patient taken any medication, alcohol or illicit drugs?

Seizure
- How did the patient behave during the event? Did this change during the event?
- Was there a loss of consciousness?
- How long did the event last?
- What happened to the eyes during the event?
- Can the patient remember 'hitting the ground'?
- Did the patient stop breathing? Did the patient bite his or her tongue?
- Was there any colour change?
- Was there any obvious injury during the event?
- Was the patient incontinent?

Post-seizure
- How was the patient immediately after the event?
- How long did it take to make a full recovery?

- When the patient recovered, were there any other symptoms remaining, e.g. weakness?
- Was there a fever present?
- Identify if there have been previous episodes. If so, assess frequency, exacerbating/relieving factors and any other neurology.

> **Clinical insight**
>
> Patients with psychological or psychiatric problems may present with functional weakness (e.g. psychosomatic). Suspect this if:
> - there is a non-anatomical distribution of the weakness
> - there is variation on repeat examination
> - the reflexes and tone are normal

Weakness

Weakness and numbness are often confused by patients. Take time to clarify what the patient understands by the symptoms that he or she reports.

Signs

Key signs are demonstrated in **Table 8.2**.

Tremor

There are several forms of tremor:
- resting tremor (e.g. Parkinson's disease)
- action tremor:
  - postural (e.g. essential tremor): occurs when maintaining a posture
  - kinetic: occurs on voluntary movements
  - intention (e.g. cerebellar lesion): occurs at end of movement
  - task specific: occurs during specific tasks such as writing
- psychogenic tremor: common, variable and distractible

Hypertonia

Hypertonia is increased tone. There are several different forms:
- **Spasticity** (or clasp-knife rigidity): hypertonia followed by a sudden 'give' on movement
- **Lead-pipe rigidity**: hypertonia throughout all movements of that joint or limb

General inspection	Abnormal gait Abnormal posture ormovements Muscle wasting or cachexia Tremor	Neurocutaneous lesions Reduced consciousness (Glasgow Coma Scale)
Eyes	Abnormal pupils Squints Ptosis	Palsy Abnormal acuity Abnormal visual fields
Speech and language	Dysarthria	Dysphasia
Face	Expressionless face Asymmetry Abnormality on ear, nose and throat exam	Neck stiffness or meningism Carotid bruits
Tone	Hypotonia Hypertonia Coordination Dysdiadochokinesia	Past pointing Abnormal heel–shin Romberg's positive
Tendon reflexes	Reduced or absent Brisk	Clonus
Abnormal sensation	Light touch Joint position sense Vibration	Pain and/or temperature

Table 8.2 Key signs on neurological examination

- **Cog-wheel rigidity**: lead-pipe rigidity associated with a tremor
- Tone and reflexes can be used to differentiate UMN and LMN lesions (**Table 8.3**)

Speech abnormalities
Speech abnormalities are discussed later in the chapter **Table 8.7**).

8.3 Neurological examination

Examination of the nervous system does not follow the same structure as other systems. There is no consensus on what the correct structure is for performing a neurological examination.

	Lower motor neurone lesion	Upper motor neurone lesion
Inspection	Wasting (atrophy of muscle) Fasciculations	No wasting
Tone	Normal or reduced	Increased (spasticity or clasp-knife)
Power	Flaccid weakness	Spastic weakness
Reflexes	Reduced or absent Downward or absent plantar	Increased tendon reflexes Upward plantar (Babinski's positive) Clonus

Table 8.3 Differentiating upper and lower motor neurone lesions

Find your own system that remains comprehensive. The following is how it is described in this chapter:
- General inspection
- Higher mental function (Chapter 10)
- Cranial nerves, including ophthalmology (Chapter 9)
- Gait
- Peripheral nervous system:
  - tone
  - power
  - reflexes
  - sensation
  - coordination
  - special tests
- Cerebellar examination

On examining the neurological system it is important to note that there is a range of normal findings, which depend on the patient, age and sex. Always compare both sides. If they differ, determine which side has the abnormality.

Positioning the patient   Wherever possible, the optimal positions for a neurological examination are:
- cranial nerves: seated
- upper limbs: seated
- lower limbs: supine

Neurology toolkit

A collection of equipment (**Figure 8.4**) is needed in order to undertake a thorough neurological examination.

Abbreviated neurological assessment

An abbreviated neurological assessment can be undertaken in approximately 5–10 minutes (**Table 8.8**). If any asymmetry or other abnormality is found then perform a full neurological examination.

8.4 Examination of the peripheral nervous system

Inspection

General inspection

With the patient adequately exposed, inspect for:
- obvious weakness
- abnormal posture or movements (**Table 8.4**)
- deformity
- tremor

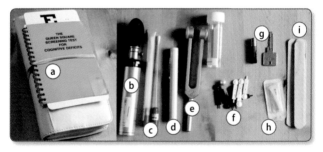

Figure 8.4 Essential equipment needed for neurological examination: (a) Snellen pocket chart for visual acuity and Ishihara plates for colour blindness; (b) ophthalmoscope for fundoscopy; (c) throat swabs for gag reflex; (d) pen-torch for pupil responses; (e) tuning forks for vibration sense testing; (f) Neurotip for pinprick testing and visual fields testing; (g) a few small objects (e.g. key, battery) for stereognosis; (h) pupil dilators (tropicamide 1%, cyclopentolate 0.5%/1%); (i) tongue depressors for gag reflex and oropharynx

Asterixis	Flapping of the hands when the arm is held in extension and the wrist is dorsiflexed
Athetoid	Serpentine like, slow and writhing movements
Atonic	Loss of tone (therefore no movement)
Bradykinesia	Slowness or lack of movements
Chorea	Rapid, purposeless, irregular and spontaneous movements
Clonus	Rapid contraction and relaxation of muscle groups
Dystonia	Contraction of agonist and antagonist muscles producing an abnormally positioned body part(s)
Fasciculations	Appear as rippling of the muscles
Myoclonus	Short and shock-like movements
Tic	Repetitive movements, suppressed for brief periods with effort or distraction
Tonus	The continuous contraction of a muscle group resulting in abnormal posture
Tremor	Repetitive, rhythmical and regular movements

Table 8.4 Involuntary and abnormal movements

- muscle wasting and fasciculations (signs of LMN lesion)
- neurocutaneous lesions

Gait

Wherever possible, perform a gait assessment. Always be ready to support a patient with weakness or balance problems. A 'get-up-and-go' test is an easy way to start (see page 321). The gait cycle is divided into stance and swing phases (**Figure 8.5**). Observe the gait from different angles (front, side and behind) with and without mobility aids (where possible):
Ask the patient to:
- remove shoes and socks
- stand from a seated position. Stand for 30 seconds (eyes open) assessing balance
- perform the Romberg's test *(see below)*
- stand on one leg, then the other

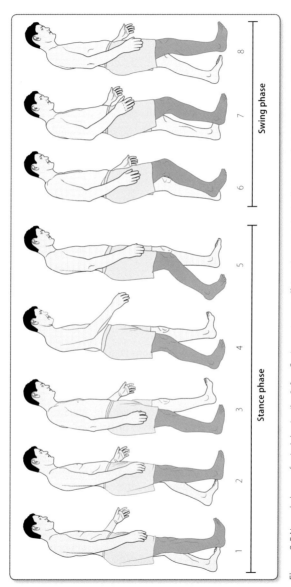

Figure 8.5 Normal phases of gait. 1, heel strike; 2, foot flat/opposite toe-off; 3, midstance; 4, heel-off/opposite foot strike; 5, toe-off; 6, foot clearance; 7, midswing/tibia vertical; 8, heel strike.

- walk to the end of the room, turn and walk back again
- walk: (1) heel to toe (imagine you are walking on a tightrope), (2) on the toes and (3) on the heels
- squat (not always necessary or possible)

Clinical insight

Gait: Observe the patient's casual gait as he or she walks into the consulting room, ideally with the patient unaware that he or she is being observed. This gives a useful comparison for formal gait assessment.

In children ask them to sit on the floor and then stand up (**Gower's test**)

As the patient undertakes each of the tests observe:
- obvious characteristic gait (**Table 8.5**)
- initiation of gait
- symmetry
- whether narrow or broad based
- each gait component: heel strike, toe-off, swing
- arm swing

Antalgic (painful)	Stance phase of gait is abnormally shortened (on affected side) relative to the swing phase
Apraxic	Rapid small steps, or with feet apparently glued to the floor
Ataxic	Broad based and unsteady
Choreiform	Hyperkinetic; irregular, jerky, involuntary movements
Diplegic	Abnormally narrow base, dragging both legs and scraping the toes Scissoring often present
Festinant	Steps have a tendency to accelerate and become faster
Hemiplegic	Extended hip and ankle that swing out to the side
Myopathic	Waddling; Trendelenburg's test positive bilaterally
Neuropathic	Seen in foot drop; high stepping, unsteady with foot slapping
Parkinsonian	Slow, shuffling gait, reduced arm swing; many steps to turn

Table 8.5 Abnormal gaits

- length and height of stride
- steadiness
- effective turn

Romberg's test

Romberg's test assesses **proprioception** (body position sense) and vestibular function (head position in space) when vision is illuminated (i.e. eyes closed). Perform as follows:

- Observe the patient's balance as he or she stands from a seated position
- In a standing position, observe balance with feet together and eyes open
- Stand behind the patient in order to give support if he or she was to become unstable
- Ask the patient to close the eyes

Romberg's test is positive if the patient becomes unsteady, sways or falls on closing the eyes. A positive Romberg's test suggests disease of the dorsal column, neuropathy or vestibular disease (e.g. alcohol intoxication). Romberg's test is not a sign of cerebellar disease. A patient with cerebellar ataxia will be unsteady even with the eyes open.

Tone

Tone is residual muscle tension created by passive partial contraction of muscles. It is vital for maintaining normal posture. It is assessed as the muscles' resistance to passive movements and can be normal, reduced (floppy, hypotonia) or increased (stiff, hypertonia). It takes experience to determine these.

To test tone, the patient needs to be exerting no voluntary control over the muscles. Ask the patient to relax the muscles as much as possible (e.g. 'Let me take the weight of your arm and let all your muscles go floppy'). Start some general conversation to distract the patient from the examination. Make serial movements of the joints at varying speeds.

Upper limbs

- Take the patient's hand as if to shake it: supinate and pronate (**Figure 8.6a**)
- Flex and extend the elbow (**Figure 8.6b**)

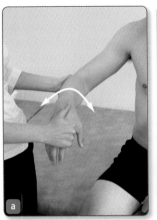
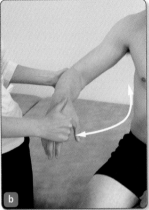
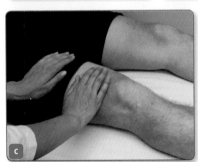
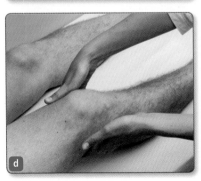

Figure 8.6 Assessing tone: (a) elbow supination/pronation, (b) elbow extension/flexion, (c) roll leg, (d) left and drop leg.

Lower limbs
- Patient supine: at the thigh, roll the leg like a log (**Figure 8.6c**)
- Rapidly lift the leg at the knee, watching the ankle (does it rise?), then drop the knee to see how quickly it falls (**Figure 8.6d**)
- If possible, repeatedly flex and extend the hip and knee in one movement

Clonus This is a series of abnormal rhythmical muscle contractions. Up to two beats of clonus are normal. Clonus is most commonly found at the ankle and is typically elicited by abrupt, sustained, hyperdorsiflexion at the ankle joint. Occasionally it can be elicited on tendon reflexes.

Power
Resistance testing Understanding these complex movements and instructions can be difficult for some patients. Resistance testing is an easy way to overcome this: place the limb at the middle of its range of movement and then ask the patient to resist your movements (e.g. 'Stop me moving your arm' – **Figures 8.7** and **8.8**). Only one movement should be tested at a time by supporting the joint above and testing below the joint (i.e. not across two joints). If abnormalities are present, additional testing will be required (to determine specific nerve or nerve root).

Describing weakness Power should be described using the Medical Research Council's (MRC's) classification of motor power:
- **Grade 0:** no movement
- **Grade 1:** flicker of movement
- **Grade 2:** can move joint with gravity eliminated
- **Grade 3:** can move joint against gravity, but not against resistance
- **Grade 4:** can move against resistance but has not got normal power
- **Grade 5:** normal power

Any weakness should be described in terms of its anatomical position, functioning movements and, if possible, nerve or nerve root distribution. Gross distributions of weakness can be described as monoparesis, hemiparesis, paraparesis or quadriparesis (**Figure 8.9**).

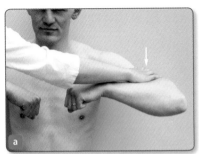

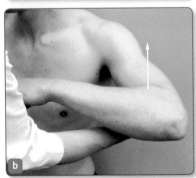

Figure 8.7 Resistance testing of power of upper limbs (arrows indicate the direction of force exerted by the examiner): (a) shoulder abduction (C5–6); (b) shoulder adduction (C5–6); (c) elbow extension (C7); (d) elbow flexion (C5–6); (e) wrist extension (C6); (f) wrist flexion; (g) grip (C8).

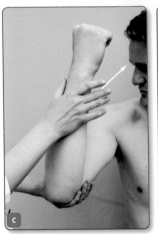

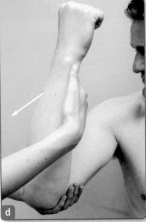

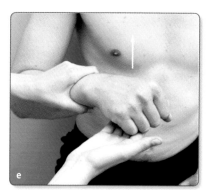

Figure 8.7 *Contd...*

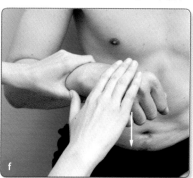

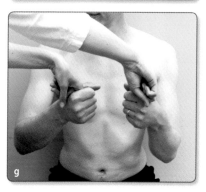

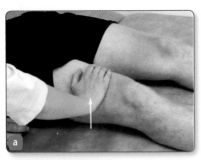

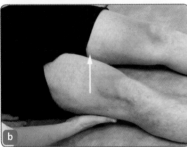

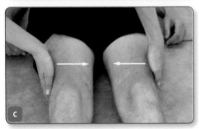

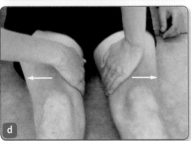

Figure 8.8 Resistance testing of lower limbs (arrows indicate the direction of force exerted by the examiner while giving the instruction 'push against me'): (a) hip flexion (L1–2); (b) hip extension (L5–S1); (c) hip abduction (L5); (d) hip adduction (L2–3); (e) knee flexion (S1); (f) knee extension (L3–4); (g) ankle plantarflexion (S1–2); (h) ankle dorsiflexion (L4).

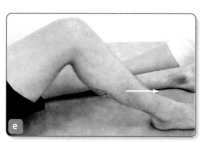

Figure 8.8 *Contd...*

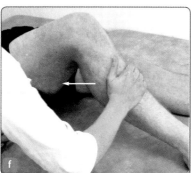

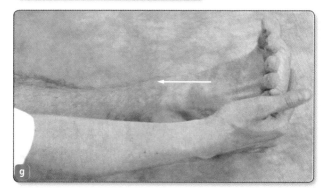

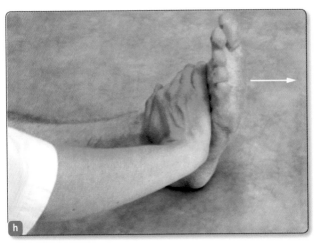

Figure 8.8 *Contd...*

Upper limb

To assess power in the upper limb, do the following:

- Place one index finger in each of the patient's palms: 'Squeeze my fingers as tightly as you can'
- Perform resistance testing (**Figure 8.7**)

Pronator drift The patient (eyes closed) should be stood upright with the arms fully extended and pronated. They should hold this posture for 5–10 seconds. Downward drift of an arm suggests a UMN lesion in the corticospinal tract.

Lower limb

Gait assessment will have revealed a great deal of information. To assess power in the lower limb, perform resistance testing (**Figure 8.8**).

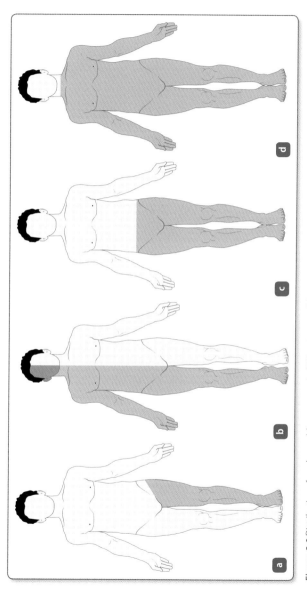

Figure 8.9 Distribution of weakness: (a) monoparesis, (b) hemiparesis, (c) paraparesis or (d) quadriparesis.

Reflexes

Similar to tone, the patient needs to relax in order to assess reflexes. Hold the tendon hammer at the end of the handle. Swing the hammer in a pendulum motion. Grade the reflex according to the response and compare sides for symmetry:

- **Grade 0:** absent
- **Grade 1:** reduced (hypoactive)
- **Grade 2:** normal
- **Grade 3:** increased (hyperactive)
- **Grade 4:** hyperactive with clonus

Reinforcement procedures If the reflex appears absent, use reinforcement procedures to identify reduced but present reflexes. These should be performed immediately before striking the tendon. For the upper limbs, ask the patient to clench his or her teeth. For the lower limbs ask the patient to clasp the hands together. He or she should try to 'pull them apart' immediately before eliciting the reflex (Jendrassik's manoeuvre).

Upper limbs

Test biceps, triceps and brachioradialis (**Figure 8.10a–8.10c**):

- Biceps (C5–6): place your thumb/finger on biceps tendon and strike your thumb
- Triceps (C7): directly strike the triceps tendon
- Brachioradialis (C5–6): either place your finger on brachioradialis or strike it directly (10 cm above the wrist on the radial aspect of the forearm)

Lower limbs

Test the patella and Achilles tendon (**Figure 8.10 d** and **8.10e**):

- Patella (knee, L2–4): flex both knees and support with one arm, directly strike the patellar tendon inferior to the patella and superior to the tibial tuberosity
- Achilles tendon (ankle, L5–S2): flex the knee and dorsiflex the ankle, supporting it on the opposing leg. Directly strike the Achilles tendon

Plantar reflex Run a blunt instrument in a J stroke up the lateral aspect of the plantar surface of the foot (**Figure 8.11**). A normal

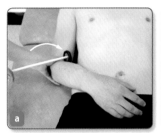
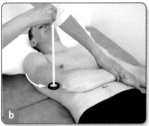
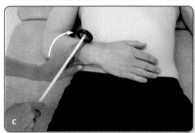

Figure 8.10 Deep tendon reflexes: (a) biceps (C5–6); (b) triceps (C7); (c) brachioradialis (C5–6); (d) patella (L2–4); (e) Achilles tendon (L5–S2).

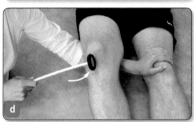

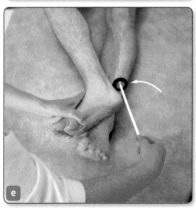

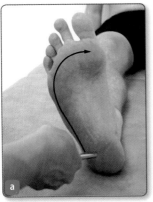
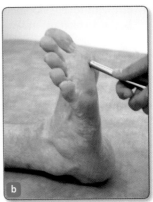
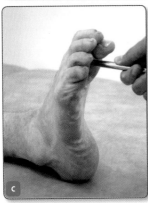

Figure 8.11 Plantar reflex: (a) method, (b) Babinski's sign positive, (c) Babinski's sign negative.

response is hallux (big toe) flexion. **Babinski's sign** is hallux extension.

Sensation

The principles of the sensory examination are to:

- start distally and work proximally
- test each major peripheral nerve
- test all the major dermatomal regions (**Figure 8.3**) bilaterally for symmetry

- test light touch, vibration, proprioception (screening the posterior columns) and lateral pain and temperature (screening the lateral columns)
- map out any area of sensory change encountered

Primary sensory modalities These test the integrity of afferent (e.g. sensory or input) sensory pathways. The patient should keep the eyes closed for all sensory testing. Lesions in the spinal cord can affect different forms of sensation so a full assessment should include the following:

Simple or light touch Use a point of cotton wool. Demonstrate to the patient the sensation (on the forehead or sternum). Do not stroke the skin. With the eyes closed, ask the patient to report 'left' or 'right' when he or she feels the cotton wool as you work through the dermatomal regions (**Figure 8.3**). Ask the patient to report if the sensation feels different on either side.

Double simultaneous stimulation is used to detect tactile extinction (also known as hemisensory inattention). Ask the patient (eyes closed) to report if he or she can feel being touched on 'the left, the right or both'. Using either your fingers or two other stimuli (e.g. cotton wool), touch corresponding points on the upper and/or lower limbs. If tactile extinction is present the patient will be able to feel touch on each side individually, but will be unable to sense being touched on both sides simultaneously.

Joint position sense (proprioception) Start at the thumb and great toe for joint position sense (**Figure 8.12**). Fix the distal aspect of the joint on the lateral and medial aspect (to avoid stimulating pressure sensation rather than sense of joint position). Demonstrate to the patient 'this is up' and 'this is down'. Starting with very small movements, move the joint. The patient (eyes closed) should be able to determine small movements. If joint position sense is abnormal, use bigger movements. If he or she still does not detect anything, move proximally until a joint is found where it remains intact.

Vibration Use a 128-Hz tuning fork. Tap the fork on a solid surface to create a vibration but not a sound. Demonstrate the

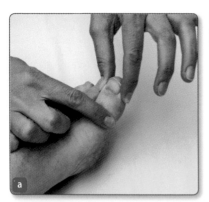

Figure 8.12 Joint position sense of the toe (a) and finger (b).

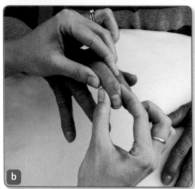

sensation on the patient's sternum. Ask the patient to report when the vibration starts. Place the non-vibrating end on the distal interphalangeal joint of the thumb. Ask the patient to report when the vibrating stops. Use your free hand to stop the vibrating end of the fork. If the patient is unable to determine vibration, move proximally along joints until he or she is able to determine vibration (**Figure 8.13**).

Pain and temperature It is necessary to test only one of these. For pain, use the sharp point of a Neurotip (medical pin). Use variations of these and ask the patient to report if he or she

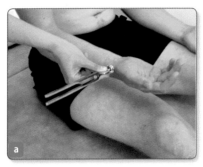

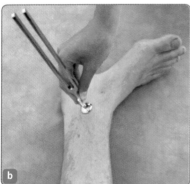

Figure 8.13 Testing for vibration sensation. (a) Upper limb: distal phalanx of the thumb > proximal end of first metacarpal > medial epicondyle of elbow > head of humerus. (b) Lower limb: distal interphalangeal joint of the great toe > lateral malleolus > tibial tuberosity > anterosuperior iliac spine.

feels a sharp or dull sensation. Work through the dermatomal regions. For temperature, use tuning forks dipped (and dried) in cold and hot water.

Discriminative sensory modalities These test the ability of the cortices to analyse and interpret sensory input. This does depend on the sensory pathways reaching the cortices being normal.

Stereognosis This is the ability to recognise an object by touch alone. Using a series of small objects (e.g. coin, key, pen, paper clip), place one at a time into the patient's palm (with eyes closed) and ask him or her to name them. Use different objects for the opposite hand.

Graphaesthesia This is the ability to recognise, by touch, writing on the skin. To test graphaesthesia, inform the patient (with eyes closed) that you are going to write a number on the hand. Use the non-indelible end of a pen to write a number between 1 and 9 on the palm of the patient's hand. Ask the patient to report the number. Repeat several times on both hands.

Point localisation Briefly touch the patient (with eyes closed). Ask the patient to immediately touch the same spot.

Two-point discrimination Use two pointed callipers. Starting at the hand touch the patient (eyes closed) at approximately 15–20 mm apart. Reduce this distance until the patient reports feeling only one point. This can be repeated on different parts of the body. Normal values for young adults are 4 mm on the hand to several centimetres on the back.

Coordination
Upper limbs
Hand movements These are best tested by demonstrating them to the patient and asking the patient to copy your movements. Observe for speed, accuracy and rhythm.
- **Finger tapping**: partially extend the fingers and thumb. Tap the tips of the fingers with the thumb from index finger to little finger and back again. Repeat with the other hand or perform simultaneosly
- **Rapid alternating movements**: rapidly pronate and supinate the wrist of the right hand on a stable level surface such as the left hand or table surface (**Figure 8.14**). Repeat with the left hand. Inability to perform this test is known as **dysdiadochokinesia**

Finger–nose test Position your own hand at an arm's length from the patient. Ask the patient to touch his or her own nose with the right hand. Ask the patient to reach out and touch the tip of your finger with the tip of his or her own finger. It is paramount that the patient's arm should achieve maximal extension and reach (**Figure 8.15**). Repeat several times, mov-

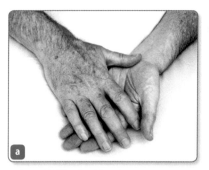

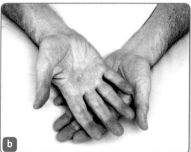

Figure 8.14 Rapid alternating movements.

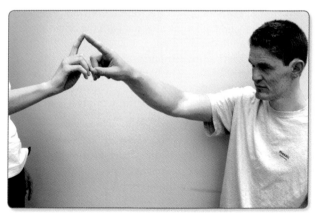

Figure 8.15 Finger–nose test.

ing the position of your finger (i.e. giving varying targets). Observe for tremor and dysmetria (overshooting or 'past pointing' the target). Repeat with the opposing hand.

Lower limbs

Heel–shin test With the patient supine ask him or her to 'Place your right heel on your left heel, now run it up to your left knee and back down again' (**Figure 8.16**). Repeat on the opposing side.

Clinical insight

The cerebellum is responsible for ipsilateral coordination and balance. To assess cerebellar function, test:

- nystagmus
- gait – including 'tight-rope walking'
- tone
- finger–nose test
- dysdiadochokinesia
- Romberg's test (patient will be unsteady with eyes open and closed)
- speech

Heel tapping Place the palm of your hand under the patient's calf. Ask the patient to use the heel to tap your palm repeatedly.

Special tests
Meningism

In certain cases an examination for meningism may need to be performed:

- **Neck (nuchal) stiffness**: patient supine; watching the hip and knees, lift the head off the bed. In a normal patient, the chin should easily touch the chest without causing neck pain
- **Brudzinski's test**: on testing neck stiffness, when meningism is present, flexing the neck causes hip and knee flexion
- **Kernig's sign**: patient supine; flex the hip and the knee to 90°. Keep the hip flexed. When meningism is present, extending (straightening) the knee causes the head to lift off the bed to release the pain

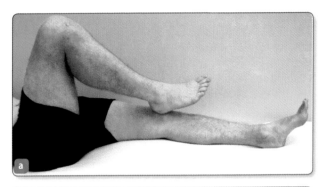

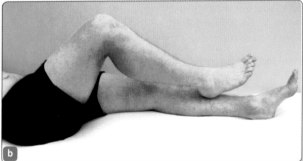

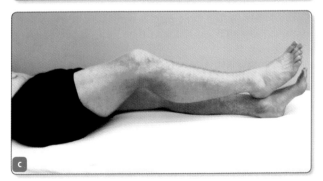

Figure 8.16 Heel–shin test (a) 'touch your knee with your heel', (b) 'run it down your shin', (c) 'and touch your ankle'.

8.5 Higher mental function

Neurology and psychiatry both frequently require an in-depth assessment of cognitive abilities. These assessments should be undertaken in a quiet room without disruption. An examination of higher mental function should include: level of consciousness, attention and concentration, memory, language, visual spatial perception, praxis and calculations.

Level of consciousness (arousal)

During the consultation it is possible to ascertain if the patient is alert, attentive, sleepy or unresponsive. The Glasgow Coma Scale (Table 15.3) is used to quantify reduced consciousness.

Language

Language is a complex process involving speech production and speech recognition (comprehension). Grossly abnormal speech (**Table 8.6**) is often evident from the start of the consultation. Be sure that the patient can hear and is functionally fluent in your own language. Speech can be grossly assessed while performing the Mini-Mental State Examination (MMSE).

Formalised assessments of higher mental function

Clock drawing

Clock drawing is used as an assessment for verbal understanding, cognitive function, spatial awareness, visual neglect and memory. It is often used as a rapid assessment of higher mental function. Give the patient a piece of blank paper and ask him or her to draw a clock face. If the patient is successful ask him or her to draw hands for a certain time.

Abbreviated mental test

The Abbreviated Mental Test (AMT) (**Table 8.7**) is a rapid screening tool for dementia/delirium (score ≤6) and is used to find patients where more extensive testing (MMSE) is required. It is acceptable to ask culturally appropriate questions for memory recall (e.g. 'When did England win the world cup?' rather than 'When was the First World War?').

Disorder	Testing	Causes
Dysphasia (expressive) Impairment of language function (also known as Brocha's aphasia)	Normal understanding (e.g. written, 'close your eyes') Unable to answer questions Unable to repeat sentences Say: 'Do you want to be able to say something but are unable to say it? Nod if yes'	Lesion to Broca's area (**Figure 8.1**)
Dysphasia (receptive) Impairment of language function (also known as Wernicke's aphasia)	Unable to understand questions or commands Speech is fluent but often meaningless Unable to repeat sentences	Lesion to Wernicke's area
Dysphasia (global) Impairment of language function	Both comprehension and speech affected	Both Broca's and Wernicke's areas affected
Dysathria Impaired or abnormal articulation of speech defective movements of lips, tongue or palate	Ask the patient to repeat the sounds: 'mmm' (lip strength, cranial nerve VII), 'KKK' (oropharnygeal muscles, cranial nerve IX and X) and 'la la la' (tongue strength, cranial nerve XII) Ask the patient to repeat the phrases: 'baby hippopotamus' and 'red lorry, yellow lorry'	Cerebellar disorders Disorder of muscles and nerves supplying jaw and mouth Extrapyramidal lesione Lower motor neuron lesion of cranial nerves
Dysphonia Impaired or abnormal sound production (volume)	Ask the patient to count from 20 down to 1 Ask the patient to say 'a, e, i, o, u'	Extrapyramidal disorders Laryngeal disease Neuromuscular weakness (e.g. myasthenia gravis) Vocal fold lesions
Dysfluency A stammer/stutter	Words are repeated, drawn out, incomplete and/or skipped	Usually developmental (i.e. during childhood)

Table 8.6 Speech abnormalities

1	How old are you?
2	What time is it (to the nearest hour)?
3	Please remember this address '42 West Street'
4	What year is it?
5	Where are you?
6	Identify two people (e.g. nurse, doctor)
7	What is your date of birth?
8	When was the First World War [or appropriate event]?
9	Who is the current president or monarch?
10	Please count backwards from 20 to 1
Ask patient to recall the address	

Table 8.7 Abbreviated Mental Test (AMT)

Orientation	In time and space
Registration	How many rounds of repetition are re for the patient to learn the names of three objects
Attention and calculation	By counting or spelling backwards
Recall	Recall of three objects learned earlier
Language and related skills	Naming an item Repeating an abstract phrase Following a simple set of spoken instructions Following written instructions Composing a full sentence Copying a the layout of simple angular drawing

Table 8.8 Summary of the mini-mental state examination (MMSE). This employs a series of pre-set questions each allocated a maximum score, to assess cognitive state. Most organisations have a preprinted version of the MMSE. The original MMSE was created by Folstein et al. (1975), J Psychiatr Res. 1975;12:189-98.

Mini-mental state examination

The MMSE (**Table 8.8**) is the most widely used cognitive test. It takes 5–10 min to complete. It tests most of the areas of higher mental function. The highest score is 30 and a score ≤24 is suggestive of delirium or dementia (25–30 normal, 21–24 mild, 10–20 moderate, <10 severe). The score should be interpreted in terms of the pre-morbid functionality of the patient, e.g. a score of 25 in a university professor is abnormal. A summary of the mental state examination is shown in **Table 8.8**.

8.6 Common investigations

Most neurological investigation is performed by specialists. Common techniques include:

- **Magnetic resonance imaging:** of the brain or spine to examine nerve tissue lesions
- **Magnetic resonance angiography:** using contrast, to assess the vasculature in cerebrovascular and neoplastic disease
- **Computed tomography:** to assess acute stroke, suspected subarachnoid haemorrhage and moderate to severe acute head injury
- **Electromyography and nerve conduction studies:** to assess peripheral nerve and muscular function to help localise lesions
- **Electroencephalography (EEG):** to categorise and monitor the electrical activity of the brain in epilepsy
- **Lumbar puncture (LP) and cerebrospinal fluid (CSF) analysis:** CSF pressure, CSF protein and glucose, microscopy, culture & sensitivity (MC&S)
- **Spinal tap and cerebrospinal fluid:** analysis to assess for inflammation in the central nervous system

8.7 System summary

An abbreviated neurological assessment is given in **Table 8.9**.

General	Wash hands; ensure privacy; introduce self and explain examination Gain consent for examination; offer a chaperone; position patient (lower limbs: patient lying down; upper limbs: patient sat up); expose area being examined
Vital signs	Temperature; pulse rate; blood pressure
Screening assessment	Upper limbs: arms out in front and palms upwards, eyes closed Lower limbs: get-up-and-go test (including gait), where possible
Higher mental function	Orientation to time, place and person; complete complicated command without non-verbal cues
Inspection	General inspection; asymmetry or deformity; posture of body
Tone	Upper limbs; lower limbs; clonus
Power	Pronator drift; grip; shoulder abduction and adduction; elbow flexion and extension; wrist flexion and extension; finger extension and abduction; thumb adduction and abduction Hip flexion and extension; hip abduction and adduction; knee flexion and extension; ankle plantar and dorsiflexion; dorsiflexion of big toe
Reflexes	Biceps and triceps; knee and ankle; plantar (Babinski's sign)
Sensation	Light touch distally in all four limbs; double simultaneous stimulation Stereognosis or graphaesthesia
Coordination	Finger tapping; finger to nose; heel–knee–shin

Table 8.9 Examination of the neurological system: an abbreviated summary

Cranial nerves and ophthalmology

Cranial nerve lesions are rare, whereas disorders of the eye are common; both can be serious. An ability to perform a slick and thorough eye and cranial nerve examination is essential. Cranial nerve examination should be included as part of a complete neurological examination (Chapter 8).

9.1 System overview

Anatomy review

Cranial nerves

The **cranial nerves** (CNs) have nuclei in the cortex and brain stem. These nerves are responsible for both motor and sensory functions (**Table 9.1**).

Motor function	Sensory function	Autonomic function
I Olfactory		
	Smell	
II Optic		
	1. Visual acuity 2. Afferent limb in pupillary response	
III Oculomotor		
1. Movements of eyes (**Figure 9.4**) 2. Elevation of eyelid		1. Pupil constriction (parasympathetic fibres) 2. Pupil dilatation (sympathetic fibres running independent of CN III)
IV Trochlear		
Inferomedial movement of eye		

Table 9.1 Cranial nerves (CNs) and functions

Contd...

Motor function	Sensory function	Autonomic function
V Trigeminal		
Muscles of mastication	1. Sensation of the face (**Figure 9.8**) 2. Cornea (corneal reflex)	
VI Abducens		
Lateral movement (abduction) of eye		
VII Facial		
1. Muscles of facial expression 2. Corneal reflex 3. Stapedius	1. Taste of anterior two-thirds of the tongue 2. External auditory meatus 3. Tympanic membrane	Salivary and lacrimal glands
VIII Vestibulocochlear		
	1. Vestibular branch – senses sound 2. Cochlear branch – sense of rotation and balance	
IX Glossopharyngeal		
	1. Taste from posterior third of the tongue 2. Sensation from palatine tonsils	Parotid gland
X Vagus		
1. Laryngeal and pharyngeal muscles 2. Muscles of the voice, resonance of the soft palate	Taste from the epiglottis	Parasympathetic fibres to thoracic and abdominal viscera

Table 9.1 *Contd...*

Contd...

Motor function	Sensory function	Autonomic function
XI Accessory		
Sternocleidomastoid and trapezius		
XII Hypoglossal		
Muscles of the tongue (important for swallowing and speech articulation)		

Table 9.1 *Contd...*

The visual tract

The visual tract (**Figure 9.1**) comprises the second cranial nerve (CN II). The eye is moved by a series of muscles that are innervated by CNs III, IV and VI (**Figure 9.2**). Understanding the innervation and anatomy of the eye is fundamental to a full ophthalmic examination (**Figure 9.3**).

9.2 Symptoms and signs

Symptoms

Visual symptoms

When assessing a patient's vision, find out whether the problem is unilateral or bilateral and identify if one of the following symptoms is present:
- the need for corrective spectacles
- ocular pain (with or without a 'red eye')
- visual disturbance:
  - double vision (diplopia)
  - blurred vision
  - sudden- or gradual-onset visual loss
  - distortion of vision
  - flashes or floaters
  - haloes

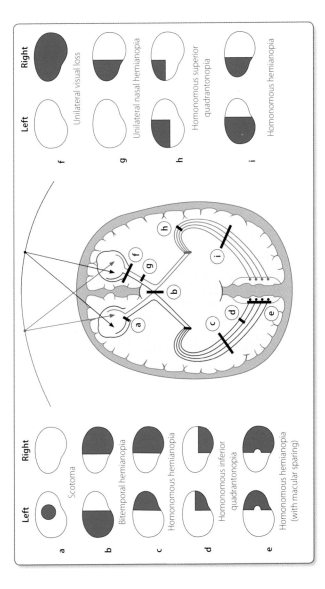

Figure 9.1 The optic tract and their relation to the visual fields.

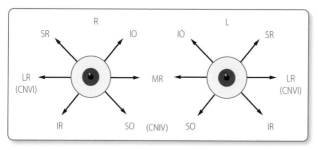

Figure 9.2 Ocular movements. SR, superior rectus; IO, inferior oblique; LR, lateral rectus; IR, inferior rectus; SO, superior oblique; MR, medial rectus.

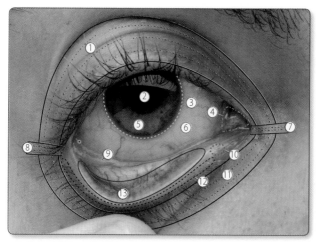

Figure 9.3 The eye and eyelid: ①, Superior tarsus; ②, pupil; ③, margin of cornea; ④, region of lacrimal lake covering lacrimal caruncle; ⑤, iris; ⑥, sclera; ⑦, medial palpebral ligament; ⑧, lateral palpebral ligament; ⑨, inferior conjunctival fornix; ⑩, lacrimal punctum on the lacrimal papilla; ⑪, inferior tarsus; ⑫, region of openings of the ciliary glands and of sty formation (black dotted line); ⑬, location of tarsal glands and of tarsal chalazion formation (red line).

– eye watering
– headaches

Ask about trauma, a family history of eye problems, systemic illness and any previous similar symptoms.

9.3 Examination of the cranial nerves

A slick, rapid examination of the cranial nerves can be under-taken in less than 10 minutes.

Cranial nerve I

Loss of smell is rarely due to a neurological condition. Test smell only if the patient reports a change. Use recognisable smells (e.g. vanilla or coffee) held in identical bottles. Test the patency of each nostril individually by occluding the other nostril and asking the patient to sniff.

Cranial nerve II (optic)

Visual acuity

Assess visual acuity with and without any corrective spectacles or a pinhole. Assess near vision formally with a Jaeger card, held 30 cm from the eyes. Ask the patient to read the smallest line possible. Distant vision is assessed for each eye individually, with a standard Snellen-type chart.

Assess in the following order, with the need for each subsequent test suggesting worsening acuity:

1. Snellen chart at 6 m: report the smallest size of letter that the patient is able to read at 6 m, e.g. 6/18 = can see size 18 letter at 6 m
2. Bring the patient forward until he or she can read the largest letter and then report the distance in metres (e.g. 2/60 = can see size 60 letter at 2 m)
3. Finger count
4. Hand movements
5. Light perception

Visual fields

Any lesion along the visual pathway can cause visual field defects (**Figure 9.1**). To assess each visual field, ask the patient to shut or occlude one eye while keeping the open eye fixed on the examiner's open eye. Use confrontation (**Figure 9.4**): ask the patient to state as soon as the movement of the fingertip is observed. Compare this with your own visual field. Assess the blind spot using a Neurotip.

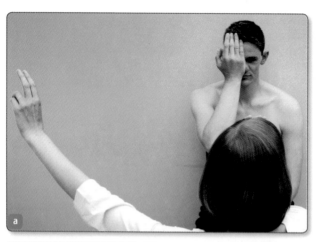

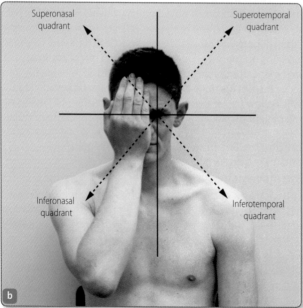

Figure 9.4 Visual fields: (a) confrontation, (b) dashed line indicates directions of movement of examiner's hand.

Assess for visual neglect and gross field defects. Ask the patient to keep both eyes open and look straight ahead. With both your arms outstretched, wiggle one and/or occasionally two fingers and ask the patient to report on which side they observed movement.

Colour vision

Use Ishihara test plates to assess colour vision in each eye independently.

Ophthalmoscopy

Having examined the undilated pupils and iris, it is best to dilate the pupils with drops (e.g. 1% tropicamide and 2.5% phenylephrine). Ophthalmoscopy should be performed in a dimly lit room. Use your right eye to examine the patient's right eye and vice versa. Place your free hand on the patient's forehead and ask the patient to fix on an object directly ahead. Change the lens to 10+ (red) and observe the red reflexes from approximately 30 cm (**Figure 9.5**). Move towards the patient until your forehead is resting on your free hand on the patient's forehead. Rotate the lens in the ophthalmoscope until the retina comes clearly into focus. Inspect the optic disc for shape, colour and vessels (**Figure 9.6**). Follow the vessels out into the four quadrants. Finally ask the patient to look at the light in order to inspect the macula.

Cranial nerves III (oculomotor), IV (trochlear) and VI (abducens)

Eye movements

Look for any immediately abnormal movements such as nystagmus. **Nystagmus** is an involuntary, rhythmic oscillation of the eyes. The movement can be horizontal, vertical, rotatory or even multidirectional.

Ask the patient to focus both eyes on an object (e.g. a finger or Neurotip) and follow the object through the six cardinal gaze positions with their eyes while

---

Clinical insight

Ophthalmoscopy: To gain the best view of the retina possible, position yourself as close to the eye as physically possible.

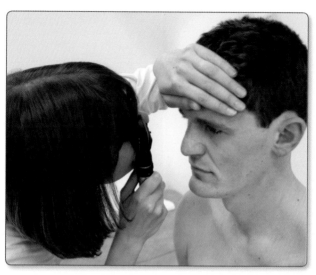

Figure 9.5 Ophthalmoscopy: examiner's right eye to patient's right eye and vice versa.

keeping the head still (**Figure 9.2**). Ask the patient to report any double vision at any point. Inspect the patient's eye movements to identify an ocular palsy. Nystagmus may often become apparent at extremes.

Assess for lid lag by asking the patient to keep the head still and follow your finger, moving centrally from the superior to an inferior position. Watch how the upper eyelid moves with the downward movement of the eye. There should be perfect coordination. If lid lag is present the upper eyelid appears to lag behind the movement of the eye.

Pupils

Pupils should be black, round, central, equally sized and reactive to light. A normal pupil size is 3–5 mm, but this depends upon the ambient lighting. Constriction (<3 mm) is known as **miosis,** whereas dilatation (>5 mm) is known as **mydriasis.** To assess the pupils, do the following:

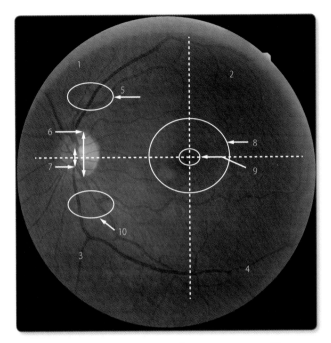

Figure 9.6 Normal retina (and quadrants). ①, supranasal quadrant; ②, supratemporal quadrant; ③, infranasal quadrant; ④, infratemporal quadrant; ⑤, superior vascular arcade; ⑥, optic disc; ⑦, optic cup; ⑧, macula; ⑨, fovea centralis; ⑩, inferior vascular arcade.

- Inspect both pupils in normal lighting then dim lighting: are they equal in size, shape and position? **Anisocoria** refers to pupils of unequal size
- Assess both the direct and indirect (consensual) light reflex. Bring the light source in from the side to avoid an accommodation reflex affecting the pupil response
- Test for accommodation: ask the patient to focus on your finger as you bring it to a position placed 30 cm from patient's nose. During this period the pupil should constrict and converge. Then ask the patient to shift the gaze to a distant object and note dilatation and divergence
- Note any abnormal pupil sizes or responses (**Table 9.2**)

Pupil type	Appearance	Features	Causes
Normal		Normal direct and indirect light reflexes	
Unilateral fixed and dilated		Unilaterally dilated pupil not responding to light	CN III palsy Cerebral herniation (e.g. mass, bleed) Trauma
Argyll Robinson pupil		Small pupil Accommodates briskly No direct/indirect light reaction	Neurosyphilis Diabetes mellitus
Homes-Adie pupil		Unilateral dilated pupil. Accomodates slowly Absent or reduced light reflex	Post viral infection Idiopathic in young females
Horner's syndrome		Unilateral small pupil Partial ptosis of lid	Congenital Neck injury Multiple sclerosis Mediastinal neoplasia
Reactive pinpoint/small		Small pupils bilaterally Reactive to light	Opiate use Organophosphate poisoning
Bilateral fixed and dilated		Dilated pupils Non-reactive to light	Coma Brain death

Table 9.2 Abnormal pupils, responses and causes

Swinging flashlight test This test can be performed to test for a **relative afferent pupillary defect** (RAPD). Shine a light source into one eye; after 1 second swing the light to the other eye and repeat back and forth. Each pupil should constrict in response to the light. If dilatation is noted in response to direct stimulation there is impaired optic nerve function, suggesting a unilateral optic neuropathy. This is an advanced test.

Cranial nerve V
Motor function

This nerve innervates pterygoid, masseter and temporalis muscles. Place your hands on the patient's mandible and ask the patient to clench the jaw. Ask the patient to move the jaw from side to side and then open the mouth against resistance. To elicit the **jaw jerk** (**Figure 9.7**), place your thumb or finger on the patient's chin. Ask the patient to keep the mouth open and relax. Strike your thumb or finger with a tendon hammer. A brisk jaw jerk suggests a bilateral upper motor neurone lesion affecting CN V. No reflex response is a normal finding.

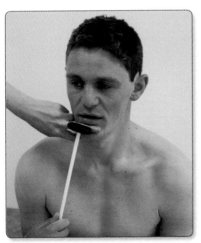

Figure 9.7 The jaw jerk.

Sensory function

Using the methods described above, test simple touch in the three distributions of the trigeminal nerve (**Figure 9.8**). **The corneal reflex** tests CN V (the **afferent,** sensory pathway) and CN VII (the **efferent,** motor pathway). Touch the cornea with a wisp of cotton wool. Both eyes should blink. This is an uncomfortable test and should not be routinely performed by a medical student.

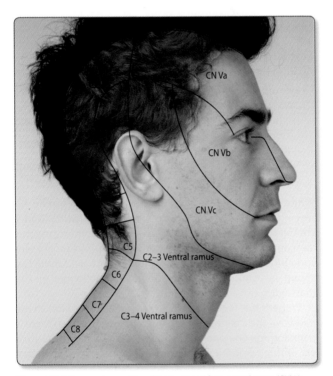

Figure 9.8 Cutaneous innervation of the head and face: cranial nerve (CN) Va, ophthalmic; CN Vb, maxillary; CN Vc, mandibular divisions.

Motor function

Ask the patient to copy facial expressions demonstrated (**Figure 9.9**). As he or she does so, inspect for any obvious asymmetry. If there is an obvious facial weakness, assess hearing because there may be a weakness in stapedius, which would result in a failure to dampen loud sounds. Look in the eyes and the mouth to assess for lacrimation and salivation respectively.

Sensory function

Use distinctive flavours (e.g. sweet, salt, bitter) to assess taste on the anterior two-thirds of the tongue.

Cranial nerve VIII

Cochlear and auditory function

Finger rub and whisper To assess hearing:

- ask the patient to close the eyes
- tell him or her to report when he or she hears a sound and on which side (left or right)
- Rub your fingers gently, close to the ear canal
- Follow this by asking the patient to repeat numbers or words whispered into the ear

Rinne's and Weber's tests Rinne's test is performed by placing a 512-Hz tuning fork on the mastoid process (bone-conducted sound) and then by the external auditory meatus (air-conducted sound) (**Figure 9.10**). In a normal ear or in sensorineural loss, the sound will be louder with air-conducted sound. In conductive loss the sound will be louder on the mastoid.

Weber's test is conducted by placing the tuning fork in the middle of the forehead. If the sound is not equal then there is pathology on one side. The sound will be louder in the normal ear, with a sensorineural deficit, and louder in the abnormal ear, with a conductive deficit.

If any deficit is identified, perform otoscopy (page 49) of the ear and organise an audiogram and tympanogram.

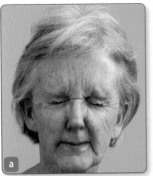
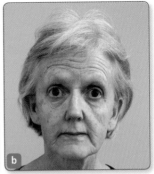
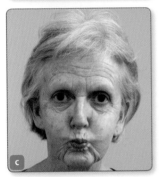
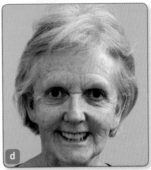
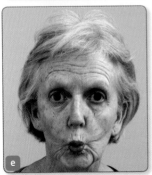

Figure 9.9 Testing muscles of facial expression: (a) 'Please close your eyes tightly'; (b) 'Please open your eyes and raise your eye brows'; (c) 'Please blow your cheeks out'; (d) 'Please smile and show me your teeth', (e) 'If you can, please whistle for me'.

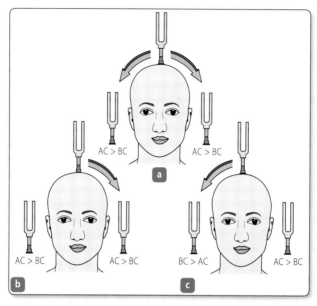

Figure 9.10 Rinne's and Weber's tests: (a) normal hearing: Weber's test is heard centrally; Rinne's test is positive on both sides, with air conduction greater than bone conduction. (b) Sensorineural deafness in the right ear: Weber's test lateralises to the better hearing (left) side; Rinne's test is positive on both sides. (c) Conductive deafness in the right ear: Weber's test lateralises to the affected right ear; Rinne's test is negative on the right side (bone conduction > air conduction) and positive on the normal left side (air conduction > bone conduction).

Vestibular function

Testing vestibular function at the bedside is difficult. To perform **Hallpike's manoeuvre** the patient is rapidly moved from a sitting position (**Figure 9.11a**) to a supine position (**Figure 9.11b**), with the head turned 45° to the right and returned to the sitting position after 20–30 s. Both sides are tested. A positive test shows nystagmus of the eye towards the affected ear when supine, with nystagmus in the opposite direction after returning to the seated position.

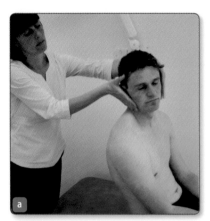

Figure 9.11 Hallpike's procedure.

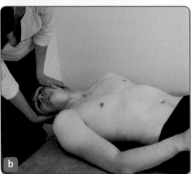

Cranial nerves IX and X
Motor function
Observe the symmetrical movements of the soft palate, uvula and posterior pharynx as the patient vocalises the sounds 'a', 'e', 'i', 'o', 'u'.

Sensory function
Touch the posterior pharyngeal wall with a tongue depressor to evoke a gag response. This tests the sensory (afferent)

function of CN IX and the motor (efferent) function of CN X. This is unpleasant so it should be performed only if a lesion is suspected. Do not routinely assess taste on the posterior third of the tongue because it is unpleasant for the patient.

Cranial nerve XI

Inspect the bulk of sternocleidomastoid and trapezius. Ask the patient to shrug the shoulders (trapezius) and rotate the head (sternocleidomastoid) against resistance.

Cranial nerve XII

Ask the patient to stick out his or her tongue and inspect it for wasting and **fasciculations** (fine, involuntary muscle contractions). A lower motor neurone lesion will cause deviation towards the affected side. Then ask the patient to push the tongue against each cheek while applying resistance.

9.4 Examination of the visual system

Eye disease is a common presentation. For a non-ophthalmologist a recommended sequence is:
1. central vision (visual acuity)
2. peripheral vision (visual fields)
3. inspection of external eye
4. eye movements
5. pupil reactions
6. cover test (if diplopia present)
7. fundoscopy

The majority of these are described above.

External eye – general inspection

Inspection should include the globe, eyelids, pupils, eyelashes, sclerae, conjunctivae and corneas.

Start by inspecting the globe for obvious lesions, trauma, asymmetry or proptosis. To assess for proptosis, inspect from the side and above the patient. Proptosis is abnormal protrusion of the eyes due to increased retro-orbital fat and oedema. On inspection, the sclera is visible above and below the iris when the eyes are open and at rest. Exophthalmos is a severe form of proptosis seen in hyperthyroidism.

Inspect the skin around the eye including the eyelids. Is the position of the lids normal? Is there any indication of ptosis (drooping of the eyelids)? Is there any periorbital or lid margin swelling/erythema?

The conjunctiva, sclera, lacrimal apparatus and cornea

Inspect the conjunctiva for inflammation, injection, follicles or papillae. Ensure that they are pink, because a pale conjunctiva can represent anaemia. Simultaneously, ensure that the sclera is not icteric (yellow – representing jaundice). If the eye is red, determine whether it is painful, unilateral, associated with a change in vision or neurological eye signs. A red eye can be caused by conjunctivitis, keratitis, episcleritis, scleritis, anterior uveitis or acute closed-angle glaucoma. Is there any abnormality in the tear ducts (lacrimal apparatus)? To visualise the cornea more accurately, one should use a yellow dye (fluorescein) and an ophthalmoscope at a +10 lens (with a cobalt blue filter).

Cover test for strabismus

A **strabismus** (also known as a **squint**) is a misalignment of the eyes. For an immediate assessment of strabismus, shine a light on the eyes from a distance of approximately 50 cm. The light should reflect symmetrically and centrally on both irises. Perform the cover test to identify if a latent or alternating strabismus (squint) is present (**Figure 9.12**). To do this:

- ask the patient to fix on your nose
- cover one eye with a card; closely observe the opposite eye
- remove the card; watch for any movement of the uncovered and covered eye
- repeat the process for the other eye
- test range of movements of eye (**Figure 9.2**) to ensure squint is not paralytic

An eye with a 'convergent squint' moves towards the midline whereas a 'divergent squint' moves away from the midline.

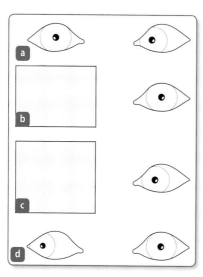

Figure 9.12 Cover test for strabismus: (a) strabismus: the visual axis of the left eye is not correctly aligned. (b) The cover test: here, as the right eye is covered (with a square card), the left eye moves to take up the gaze on the object. This is an alternating squint. (c) Here, when the good eye is covered, the left eye does not take up the gaze. This is a non-alternating squint. (d) As the right eye is uncovered the left eye remains fixed. This is an alternating (divergent) squint.

Any squint in young children needs specialist assessment because an untreated condition could lead to cortical blindness (**amblyopia**).

Completing the examination
Anterior and posterior segments
An ophthalmologist would complete the examination of the visual system by examining the anterior and posterior segments of the eyes using a slit-lamp and direct ophthalmoscopy.

9.5 Common investigations

Ophthalmological investigation is generally a specialist reserve. The following may be indicated:

- **Blood pressure:** if there are signs of hypertensive retinopathy; blood sugar and urinalysis in patients with diabetic retinopathy
- **Brain MRI:** in optic neuritis, to assess for multiple sclerosis
- **Ultrasound:** to assess the structure of the eye

- **Optical coherence tomography:** to assess tissue morphology, for example damage caused by glaucoma, multiple sclerosis, macular degeneration or retinal vessel disease
- **Fundus fluorescein angiography:** to assess retinal blood supply in diabetic retinopathy or age-related macular degeneration
- **Automated visual field testing (perimetry):** to quantify visual field defects
- **Tonometry:** to measure intraocular pressure in glaucoma
- **Gonioscopy:** uses a special lens and slit lamp to microscopically view the iridocorneal angle and whether it is blocked in glaucoma
- **Topical fluorescein:** is used to examine for corneal erosions/integrity

See page 194 for a discussion of neurological investigations.

9.6 System summary

A summary of the cranial nerve examination is given in **Table 9.3**.

General	Wash hands; ensure privacy; introduce self and explain examination Gain consent for examination; offer a chaperone; position patient (upright)
I – olfactory	Sense of smell
II – optic	Visual acuity (Snellen chart); visual fields (including the blind spot) Fundoscopy (assess the optic disc, vessels and macula) Colour vision (Ishihara chart)
III, IV and VI – oculomotor, trochlear, abducens	Range of eye movements; nystagmus Accommodation reflex; pupillary reflexes (direct and indirect) Swinging flashlight test
V – trigeminal	Muscles of mastication; sensation in each division Corneal reflex; jaw jerk (explaining procedure to patient)

Table 9.3 Examination of the cranial nerves: a summary

VII – facial	Ask the patient to raise their eyebrows and close their eyes tight, show their teeth, blow out their cheeks and whistle
	Taste on anterior two-thirds of tongue (rarely tested, but say that you would like to in exam)
VIII – vestibulocochlear	Hearing (whispering); Rinne's and Weber's tests; otoscopy to inspect ear drums
IX and X – glossopharyngeal and vagus	Gag reflex; ask the patient to say 'Aah' (look for uvular and palatal deviation)
	Taste on the posterior third of the tongue (rarely tested)
	Ask patient to speak and cough
	Inspect for adequate salivation
XI – accessory	Ask the patient to 'Shrug both shoulders' (against resistance) and 'Turn your head against my hand' – sternocleidomastoid (contralateral side)
XII – hypoglossal	Inspection of tongue for wasting, fasciculation or tremor
	Ask the patient to 'Stick your tongue out' (deviates towards paralysed side)
To finish	Full examination of the peripheral nervous system if any abnormalities found
	Higher centres and speech
	Thank and cover the patient, and wash your hands

Table 9.3 *Contd...*

Musculoskeletal system

The musculoskeletal system comprises the muscles, bones and joints. Together these are responsible for movement, breathing, maintaining body shape, protecting vital organs and storing minerals. Within the discipline of rheumatology, systemic signs are common. This chapter focuses on how to examine the bones and joints of the body.

10.1 System overview

Anatomy review
Skeletal system
The skeleton consists of bones and cartilage held together by fibrous ligaments.

Joints
A joint is the point at which two bones meet. There are three types:
1. Fixed or fibrous (e.g. skull)
2. Cartilaginous (e.g. vertebral joints)
3. Synovial (e.g. knee)

10.2 Symptoms and signs

Take a full history (**Table 10.1**) using the mnemonic OPERATES+ (Table 1.2) for each presenting complaint or problem. For each symptom clarify the effect of exercise and/or movement, whether the symptom is worse at the start or end of the day and whether there are any associated symptoms (e.g. fever).

Symptoms
Pain
Pain can arise from joints (arthralgia), muscles (myalgia) or other soft tissues. Take a pain history using the mnemonic SOCRATES (Table 1.3). Pain can be referred from joints to the surrounding

tissues or other joints (**Figure 10.1**), so always examine above and below any painful joint. Joint pain should be defined by the number of joints affected (with possible causes in brackets): **monoarticular**, one joint (trauma); **oligoarticular**, two to four joints (reactive arthritis) and **polyarticular**, five or more joints (rheumatoid arthritis).

History component	Key points
Presenting complaint	Joint pain or swelling Weakness Change in mobility Stiffness Functional deficit Numbness or paraesthesia Mechanical symptoms: clicking, locking, popping, grating from joint Inflammatory symptoms: redness, warmth
Past medical history	Previous injuries, cancers or radiotherapy Inflammatory bowel disease Eye conditions (e.g. iritis) Skin conditions (e.g. psoriasis)
Past surgical history	Joint procedures or injections
Drug history	Analgesia: paracetamol, opiates, non-steroidal anti-inflammatory diseases (NSAIDs) Steroids Disease-modifying anti-rheumatic drugs (DMARDs), e.g. methotrexate, infliximab Alternative therapies or over-the-counter medications
Family history	Joint disease, inflammatory arthropathies, e.g. rheumatoid disease, psoriasis), ankylosing spondylitis, gout/pseudogout, lupus
Social history	Ask about current or previous tobacco use (Chapter 1) Activities of daily living (ADL) – Table 1.5 – and any home adaptations Occupation or previous occupation Take a sexual history where appropriate (in suspected Reiter's syndrome or reactive arthritis)

Table 10.1 The musculoskeletal history

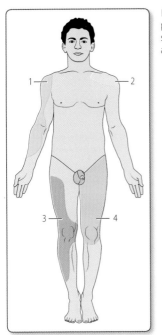

Figure 10.1 Distribution of pain arising from the joints: (1) scapulohumeral, (2) sternoclavicular/acromioclavicular, (3) knee, (4) hip.

Joint stiffness

Stiffness is subjective, so clarify what the patient means by it. Some consider it to be a loss of range of movement, others as a difficulty, or even inability, to effectively move a joint. Identify whether there is any timing to the stiffness: early morning stiffness is typically seen in inflammatory conditions such as rheumatoid arthritis, whereas evening stiffness is seen in mechanical joint disease such as osteoarthritis (**Table 10.2**).

Loss of function

Loss of function is the inability to perform a particular action.

> ## Clinical insight
>
> Red flags in musculoskeletal disease are:
> - pain with weight loss
> - unremitting, progressive, severe pain
> - pain waking the patient from sleep

Features	Rheumatoid arthritis	Osteoarthritis
Classic joint distribution	Polyarticular, often symmetrical	Mono- or oligoarthritis, non-symmetrical
Classic joint involvement	Small joints (hands and feet)	Large joints (hip and knee), spine and hands
Joint symptoms	Heat, redness, swelling and pain Stiffness in morning or after rest (relieved after several hours)	Pain worst after exercise and relieved by rest Stiffness in morning or after rest (relieved after 30 minutes) or evening stiffness
Common hand deformities	Ulnar deviation Swan-neck deformity Boutonnière's deformity Z deformities of thumbs	Bouchard's nodes Heberden's nodes
Other deformities	Feet signs, e.g. collapse of longitudinal arch Atlantoaxial subluxation in cervical spine	Valgus or varus deformities Tilting of the pelvis
Other signs	Muscle wasting and tendon rupture	Muscle wasting, crepitus, tilting of the pelvis
Systemic symptoms	Constitutional symptoms, e.g. fever, fatigue Systemic disease involvement common, e.g. anaemia, pulmonary fibrosis, scleritis	Absence of constitutional symptoms or systemic disease

Table 10.2 Signs and symptoms in rheumatoid arthritis and osteoarthritis.

This can be reported by patients either descriptively (e.g. 'I can't lift my leg') or as an inability to perform a certain task (e.g. 'I can't unlock the door'). In assessing loss of function one needs to understand the joints and actions involved in key activities of daily living (page 10).

Signs
Joint swelling and pain
If a patient reports swelling or if you find it clinically you should determine the following:

- Which joints are affected?
- Is the swelling symmetrical?
- Does the severity and timing of the swelling fluctuate?
- Is there any associated erythema or temperature change of the affected joint?
- Are there any systemic features, e.g. fever, weight loss?

Effusions

An effusion can occur in any joint secondary to trauma, inflammation or infection. They are more obvious in the superficial joints (knee, ankle, wrist or fingers) than the deep joints (shoulder or hip). It is difficult to diagnose an effusion in most joints (except the knee), and usually an ultrasound or trial aspiration is needed to confirm its presence.

Other clinical signs found in musculoskeletal examination

There are a number of classic signs found in musculoskeletal disease (**Table 10.3**).

10.3 Examination of the musculoskeletal system

The examination of each joint follows a standard format (**Table 10.7**):

- inspection (look)
- palpation (feel)
- range of movement (move): active and passive
- measurements
- special tests
- neurological and vascular examination

Before examining a particular joint it is useful to perform a GALS assessment. If the patient is in pain then take this into consideration when examining or moving him or her.

GALS assessment

The GALS (gait, arms, legs, spine) assessment is a rapid screening tool/examination for detecting musculoskeletal disorders; it can be completed in under 5 minutes. A more comprehensive

General	Lymphadenopathy Trendelenburg's test positive Abnormal gait or limp	Signs of inflammatory bowel disease
Vital signs	Fever	
Skin	Psoriasis Vasculitis	Erythema nodosum Gout
Eyes	Pallor Episcleritis Iritis	Conjunctivitis Keratitis
Neck	Pain Reduced movement	Deformity
Chest	Cervical rib	Shortness of breath
Spine	Scoliosis Thoracic kyphosis	Lumbar lordosis Reduced range of motion
Hands	Joint swelling Deformities	Nodes Muscle wasting
Face	Mouth ulcers or telangiectasia Dry mouth Parotid swelling	Pallor Butterfly rash
Joints	Reduced range of motion Swelling Pain	Inflammation Enlarged bursa Nodules
Muscles	Wasting Weakness	Tenderness
Bones	Fractures Localised tenderness	'Lumps and bumps'

Table 10.3 Key signs on musculoskeletal and rheumatological examination

examination should be performed of diseased joints identified during GALS:

History

- Do you have any pain or stiffness in your muscles, joints or back?
- Can you dress yourself completely without difficulty or help?
- Can you walk up and down stairs without difficulty?

Gait

- Watch the patient walk with or without aids as required:
    - inspect from behind, in front and the side
    - observe the patient turning

Arms

- Inspect for muscle wasting and/or joint deformity
- Active movements:
    - place both hands behind the head with elbows back (shoulder function)
    - place both arms straight out in front (elbow function)
    - put hand between shoulder blades (shoulder external rotation)
    - tuck elbows into sides; supinate then pronate hands (forearm rotation)
    - make a tight fist; examiner should assess grip strength
    - make a prayer sign (wrist flexion and finger extension) (**Figure 10.2**)
    - touch tips of each finger to the ipsilateral thumb (fine motor).

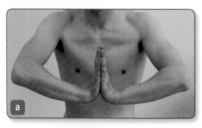
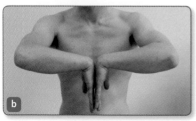

Figure 10.2 Prayer sign and reverse prayer sign.

- Examiner squeezes across the metacarpals (elicits tenderness)

Legs With the patient standing:
- inspect for swelling, deformity, leg length discrepancy

With the patient on a couch:
- feel knee for warmth
- check passive movements:
  - flex hip and knee to 90° while feeling the knee for crepitus
  - in that position rotate the hip looking for pain or stiffness
- squeeze across the metatarsals (elicits tenderness)
- inspect soles of feet for callosities or ulcers
- palpate for effusion (bulge test and patellar tap)

Spine With patient standing inspect from behind:
- Look for abnormal symmetry of shoulders, spine and hips (**Figure 10.3**)
- Confirm that head lies above the pelvis
- Deep palpation of supraspinatus, looking for **hyperalgesia** (increased sensitivity to pain)

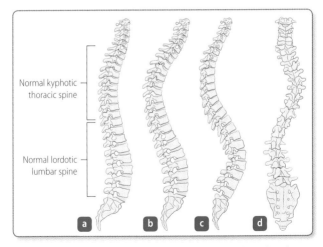

Normal kyphotic thoracic spine

Normal lordotic lumbar spine

a   b   c   d

Figure 10.3 Spinal anomalies: (a) normal; (b) kyphosis; (c) lordosis; (d) scoliosis.

With patient standing inspect from the side:
- Examine for abnormal kyphosis or lordosis
- Ask the patient to bend forward to touch the toes

With patient standing inspect from the front:
- Ask the patient to touch the ipsilateral shoulder with his or her ear
- Ask the patient to look left and look right

Joint-specific examinations

Once the GALS assessment has been undertaken, the affected joint should be examined using the look–feel–move description given below. Each joint will have some have some joint-specific requirements for the examination (**Tables 10.4** and **10.5**).

Structure to joint examination

Inspection (look)

The joint being examined should be appropriately exposed. Where possible it is best practice to simultaneously expose above and below the joint. Inspect the right and left limbs together to allow comparison. Inspection should be undertaken from the front, back and side of the patient. Take particular note of any deformities (**Table 10.6**). To inspect and palpate the hands it can be helpful to position them on a cushion (**Figure 10.4**). Inspection of the joint and surrounding tissues should identify:

- scars
- abnormal posture of the joint
- deformities (e.g. joint malalignment, fracture)
- guarding (i.e. protecting the joint); this is particularly important in children or non-verbal adults
- swelling
- inflammation or erythema
- bruising
- obvious effusions
- dermatological disease

Palpation (feel)

Observe the patient's face for signs of pain. Feel the

> ## Clinical insight
>
> A valgus deformity is one in which the distal section of a limb deviates away from the patient's midline. Varus deformity describes deviation towards the midline.

	Inspection (look)	Palpation (feel)	Movement (move) – active and passive	Special tests
Neck and spine	Torticollis Hyperextension of neck Scoliosis Kyphosis Lordosis	Midline tenderness of vertebral bodies	Extension Flexion Lateral rotation Lateral flexion Passive movements not indicated	None
Shoulder	Contour Deltoid muscle wasting Winging of the scapulae Clavicle and acromion alignment	Localised tenderness	Flexion Extension Abduction Internal rotation External rotation	Assess joint stability (stressing) Assess power in deltoid, serratus anterior and pectoralis major
Elbow	Gunstock (varus) deformity Effusion Osteophytes	Tenderness Osteophytes	Extension Flexion	Test the median, radial and ulnar nerves
Wrist	Deformities Swellings of tendon sheath	Tenderness over the radial or ulnar area	Dorsiflexion (extension) Palmar flexion (flexion)	Phalen's test Tinel's sign Durkin's test
Hand	Bouchard's nodes Boutonnière's deformity Dropped finger Heberden's nodes Mallet finger Swan-neck deformity Trigger finger	Tenderness over anatomical snuffbox Palpation of interphalangeal joints (metacarpals for swellings or tenderness)	Extension Flexion Opposing movements of thumb	Pressure along finger axis to test stability of metacarpals and phalanges

Table 10.4 Examination of the upper limb and spine

bony and soft-tissue anatomy of the relevant joint to elicit tenderness. Try to establish exactly what is under your finger when palpating the joint.

Use warm hands to palpate the joint for:

- joint temperature (compare with opposite side)

	Inspection (look)	Palpation (feel)	Movement (move) – active and passive	Special tests
Hip	Inspect gait Position of limb	Greater trochanter pain	Abduction Adduction Flexion Internal rotation External rotation	True and apparent leg lengths
Knee	Genu valgum or varum Quadriceps wasting Effusion Swelling	Tenderness Effusions	Extension Flexion	Joint effusion Joint stability Meniscal tear
Ankle	Hypertrophied calf	Swelling of tenosynovitis	Dorsiflexion Plantar flexion Inversion Eversion Medial movements Lateral movements	Joint stability of the ankle
Foot	Club foot Loss of medial arch Claw toes Hammer toes Hallux valgus or rigidus Bunions	Gout	Extension Flexion	

Table 10.5 Examination of the lower limb

	Sign	
Spine and neck	Torticollis	A 'twisted neck'; in most cases the head is tipped to one side with the chin rotated towards the opposing side
	Scoliosis	Fixed, lateral deviation of a normally straight, vertical spine (**Figure 10.16**)
	Hyperkyphosis	Exaggeration of the normal anterior facing concave curvature (kyphosis, normal range 20–50°) of the thoracic spine
	Lordosis	The normal curvature of the lumbar (normal range 20–80°) and cervical spine (normal range 20–40°) but the term is often used to describe abnormally increased curvature of these regions
Upper limb	Winging of the scapula	Protrusion of the scapula in an abnormal position
	Gunstock/varus deformity	Mal-union of a previous supracondylar fracture of the elbow
Hand/wrist	Bouchard's nodes	Osteoarthritic enlargement of the proximal interphalangeal (PIP) joints
	Boutonnière's deformity	Flexion of the PIP joints with hyperextension of the distal interphalangeal (DIP) joints
	Dropped finger (mallet finger)	Persistent flexion of the DIP joint caused by loss of extensor tendon continuity
	Heberden's nodes	Osteoarthritic enlargement of the DIP joints
	Swann-neck deformity	Extension at the PIP and flexion at the DIP joints
	Trigger finger (stenosing tenosynovitis)	Difficulty flexing and/or extending a finger (or thumb) with 'triggering' (catching, snapping or locking)
Lower limb	External rotation	Noted in hip fracture

Table 10.6 Deformities found in musculoskeletal examination

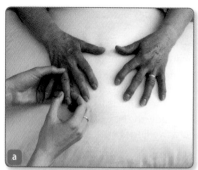

Figure 10.4 Palpation: (a) interphalangeal joints, (b) wrist joints.

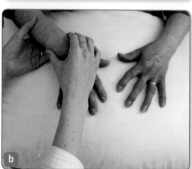

- swelling: is it bony or soft tissue?
- tenderness: describe anatomical location and severity
- crepitus ('creaking') on movement of the joint
- **osteophytes** (bony outgrowths found at joints in osteoarthritis)

If a joint is swollen, it is important to determine if the swelling is:

- hard: suggesting a bony deformity (e.g. osteoarthritis)
- fluctuant: suggesting an effusion
- soft and spongy: suggesting synovial thickening (e.g. rheumatoid arthritis)

Measurements There are a series of measures that may be required using a tape measure:
- **True and apparent leg lengths**: in a supine, straight patient, measure from the greater trochanter (true) and umbilicus (apparent) to the medial malleolus (**Figure 10.5**)
- **Calf and thigh circumference**: use a tape measure to measure the calf and thigh at the same distance on each leg for comparison above and below the knee. This provides useful information on possible swelling (increased circumference) or muscle wasting (reduced circumference)
- **Arm span (reach)**: abduct the shoulders to 90° and measure the distance between the tips of the middle fingers. A normal arm span in adults is approximately 5 cm greater than the person's height. An arm span greater than this can indicate Marfan's syndrome or age-related height loss

Range of movement (move)
Warn the patient that you will be moving the joints. Each joint has a normal range of movement.

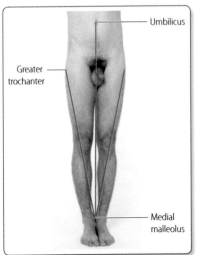

Umbilicus

Greater
trochanter

Medial
malleolus

Figure 10.5 True (blue) and apparent (red) leg lengths.

Active movements These are movements undertaken by the patient. You should assess a full range of active movements of the spine, neck, upper limbs and lower limbs (**Figures 10.6–10.16**) by asking the patient to copy your own movements or giving a series of instructions. The movements of the upper limbs can be assessed simultaneously and should be symmetrical. Reduced active movements can be classified into painful or painless. Painful reduction in movement can be caused by joint inflammation, infection or inflammatory muscular conditions (i.e. myositis). Painless reduction in movement might be secondary to weakness, spasticity or contractures. In the presence of significant joint destruction on radiography, the patient may still have little pain and a full range of movement. You may be required to assess the power of muscle groups (page 174).

Passive movements These are movements undertaken by the clinician. You should assess all the movements of the joint that you are examining. Move any painful joints last. Always watch the patient's face for signs of pain.

Joint stability Assess joint stability by applying appropriate pressure (straining), e.g. the assessment of the knee includes valgus and varus pressure to check the integrity of the collateral ligaments. To gain an accurate assessment, the muscle groups surrounding the joint must be relaxed.

Clinical insight

When describing restricted movements, they should be described as 'lacking the last x degrees', e.g. an elbow that moves 20–165° 'lacks the last 20° of extension'. A good guide is to think about your own range of movement (which is usually normal).

Clinical insight

You should initially be supervised when straining joints to avoid the possibility of causing injury.

Measure

Goniometer This is used to accurately assess the range of passive and active movements. A goniometer is a hinged rod with a protractor at the centre. Measure the joint in maximal extension and describe the movement in degrees of flexion from extension.

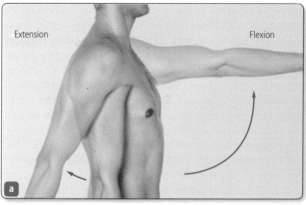

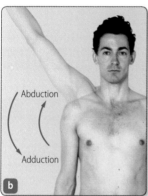

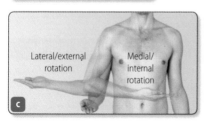

Figure 10.6 Shoulder movements: (a) Extension/flexion (no ranges); (b) abduction (180–195°); (c) external rotation (45–60°) internal rotation (>90°).

Special tests

Spine

Schober's test   With the patient standing, find L5 at the level of the iliac crests. Either mark the skin or place a finger 5 cm below and 10 cm above L5. Ask the patient to touch the toes (flexion of the spine) without bending (flexing) the knees. If the distance between the markers increases less than 5 cm then lumbar flexion is limited.

Straight leg raise/sciatic nerve stretch test With the patient in the supine position and the legs straight, flex the leg at the hip to 90° (**Figure 10.17**). Then dorsiflex the foot (**Bragard's test**). A positive stretch test occurs when pain is felt at the back of the thigh (increased further by dorsiflexion). This indicates irritation of the nerve roots supplying the sciatic nerve (L5–S2), often due to a prolapsed disc. The pain is relieved on knee flexion.

Femoral nerve stretch test   A positive femoral nerve stretch test (FNST) suggests L2–4 disc protrusions. With the patient prone (**Figure 10.18**) passively flex the knee and then extend the hip. If positive, the patient will experience anterior thigh pain.

Wrist

Carpal tunnel assessment To assess for a median nerve compression at the carpal tunnel the following will produce symptoms of numbness and tingling in the radial three and a half digits:

- **Phalen's test**: position the hands in the reverse prayer position (**Figure 10.2**) for 30–60 seconds

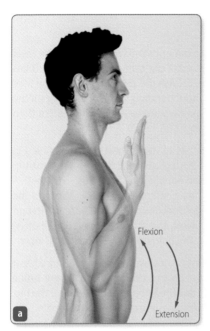

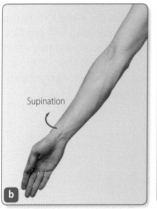

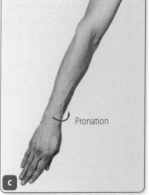

Figure 10.7 Elbow movements: (a) Flexion (145°) extension (0°); (b) pronation (70–75°); (c) supination (80–85°).

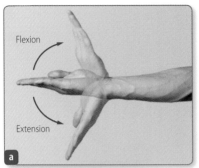

Figure 10.8 Wrist movements: (a) Extension/ flexion (70–75°); (b) abduction/adduction.

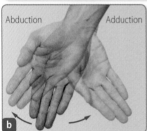

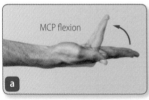

Figure 10.9 Hand movements: (a) MCP flexion (90°); (b) finger adduction; (c) finger abduction.

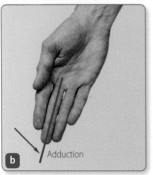

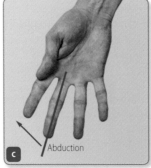

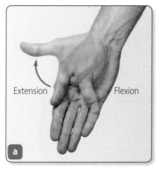

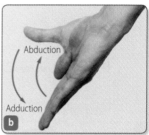

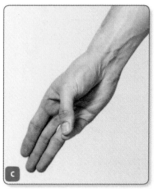

Figure 10.10 Thumb movements: (a) Extension/flexion; (b) Adduction/abduction; (c) Thumb opposition (anterior view).

- **Tinel's sign**: gentle, repetitive percussion over the median nerve at the palmaris longus tendon at the level of the distal wrist crease
- **Durkan's compression**: sustained compression over the carpal tunnel with the examiner's thumb. Positive if symptoms at 30 seconds

Hip

Trendelenburg's test Inspect from behind the standing patient. To assess the abductor muscle of the left leg, ask the patient to raise the right leg so that he or she is standing on the left leg. The pelvis should remain level or rise slightly on

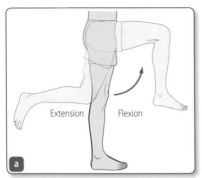

Figure 10.11 Hip movements: (a) Flexion (115–120°); (b) abduction (45–50°) and adduction (25–30°).

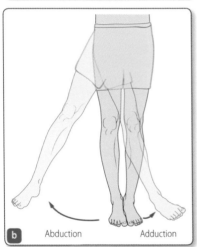

the raised leg. If the pelvis drops on the side of the raised leg then there is an abductor muscle weakness in the standing leg. Repeat on the opposite side.

Thomas's test This is used to rule out a hip flexion contracture. To examine the right leg, place your left hand under the lumbar spine while the patient lies supine. Fully flex the right hip. If the left hip lifts off the couch, there is a left fixed flexion deformity. Repeat on the left side with opposite hands.

Knee

Joint effusion Fluid is 'milked' distally from the suprapatellar pouch (**Figure 10.19a**). If fluid is present then there will be palpable bulging adjacent to the patellar tendon. After this the patella can be balloted (patellar tap) (**Figure 10.19b**).

Joint stability To assess stability of the **medial and lateral collateral ligaments,** place the lower limb in full extension and

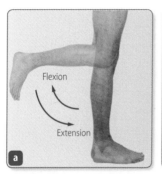
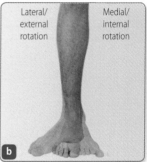

Figure 10.12 Leg movements: (a) Extension (0–5°) flexion (135–145°); (b) knee rotation.

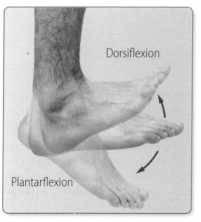

Figure 10.13 Ankle plantarflexion (45–55°) and dorsiflexion (15–20°).

stress the joint laterally and medially (**Figure 10.20**). Repeat with the joint at 20° flexion.

To assess the **cruciate ligaments,** do the following:

1. Draw's test: flex the knee to 90° with the patient lying supine. Sit on the edge of the couch and place the patient's foot under your own buttock. Ensure that the patient's hamstring is relaxed and then pull the tibia towards you (**Figure 10.21a**).

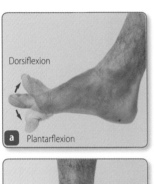

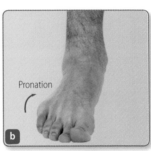

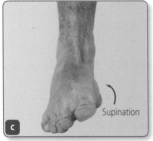

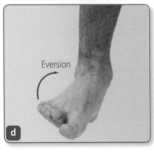

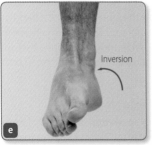

Figure 10.14 Toe movements: (a) Dorsiflexion/plantarflexion; (b) pronation; (c) supination; (d) eversion (15–20°); (e) inversion (35°).

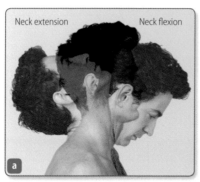

Neck extension   Neck flexion

Figure 10.15 Neck movements: (a) Extension (60°) flexion (50°); (b) Lateral flexion (45°).

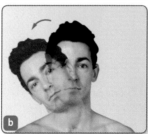

Excessive anterior displacement indicates anterior cruciate damage

2. Lachman's test: flex the knee to 30° and stabilise the distal femur with one hand. With the other hand, pull on the proximal tibia anteriorly (**Figure 10.21b**)

Meniscal tear To test for a meniscal tear perform **McMurray's test**: with the patient supine, flex the knee and place a hand on the medial side of the knee you are testing. Externally rotate the leg and bring the knee into extension. A positive test will result in a pop or click. This test should only be performed once as it can be painful.

Neurological and vascular examination

A complete musculoskeletal examination should include a neurological (Chapter 8) and vascular (Chapter 3) examination

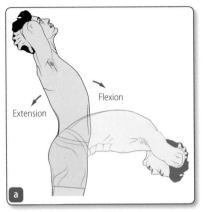

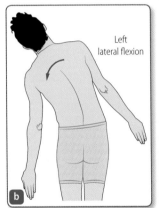

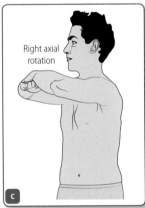

Figure 10.16 Spine movements: (a) Extension/flexion; (b) left lateral flexion; (c) right axial rotation.

of the affected limb, in particular distal to the joint being examined.

10.4 Common investigations

Common investigations of the musculoskeletal system include blood, urine and effusion fluid analysis, imaging and nerve studies.

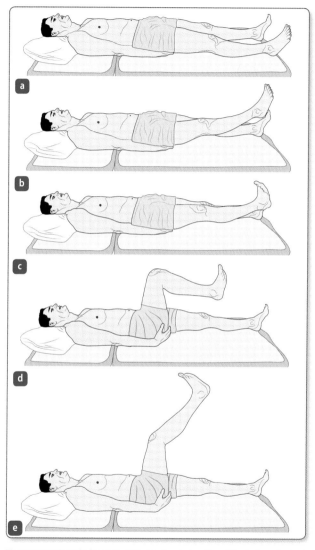

Figure 10.17 Straight-leg raise: (a) supine/neutral position; (b) raise leg – limited by pain caused by tension of root over prolapsed disc; (c) Bragard's test – pain increased by dorsiflexing foot; (d) flexion of knee relieves pain; (e) Laseque's test – extension of knee increases pain.

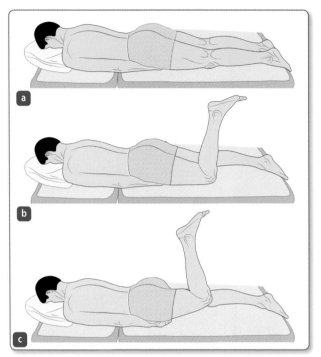

Figure 10.18 Femoral stretch: (a) patient prone and neutral (no pain); (b) pain elicited on knee flexion alone; (c) pain elicited on knee flexion and hip extension.

- **Blood tests**: full blood count (signs of inflammation or abnormal blood cells), C-reactive protein and erythrocyte sedimentation rate (raised in inflammation and infection), calcium and phosphorus (deranged in rickets, osteomalacia and parathyroid disease), alkaline phosphatase (raised in active rickets; reduced in some anaemias and bone tumours)
- **Bence-Jones protein**: found in the urine in multiple myeloma
- **Joint aspiration:** to detect crystals and infection
- **Radiography:** usually two views of the affected area, and including the joints above and below in fractures

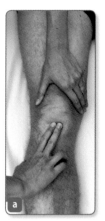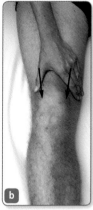

Figure 10.19 Patellar tap

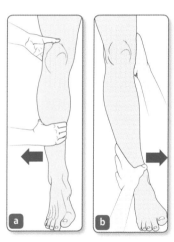

Figure 10.20 Collateral ligament stability: (a) medial stress, (b) lateral stress.

- **CT scanning:** to examine bony lesions or suspected occult fractures (not seen on radiography)
- **Ultrasound of swollen joints:** to assess which tissue is swollen and to what extent

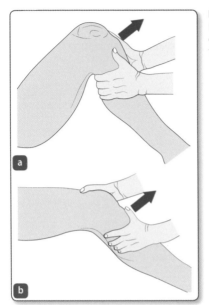

Figure 10.21 Cruciate ligaments: (a) anterior draw test; (b) Lachman's test.

- **Magnetic resonance imaging (MRI):** to assess soft tissue pathology in detail, e.g. soft-tissue knee injury or tumour staging
- **Dual-energy X-ray absorptiometry (DEXA):** to quantify bone density in osteoporosis
- **Nerve conduction studies:** to assess peripheral neuropathy due to musculoskeletal disease, e.g. in carpal tunnel syndrome

10.5 System summary

A summary of the musculoskeletal examination is given in **Table 10.7**.

Preparation	Wash hands; ensure privacy; introduce self and explain examination Gain consent for examination; offer a chaperone Position patient and expose area being examined
General inspection	Walking aids, orthoses or shoes Obvious deformity of limbs or spine in standing or lying position Observe posture and gait (spine, pelvis, lower limb)
GALS	Gait; arms; legs; spine
Focused inspection of joint/limb	Scars, inflammation or skin changes Posture, swelling or deformity of joint; muscle wasting; guarding
Joint palpation	Temperature; swelling; tenderness; crepitus; effusions; joint stability
Movement	Active movements; passive movements; assessment for pain; range of movement
Measure (where appropriate)	Goniometer Leg length: true and apparent Arm span
Special tests (where appropriate)	Calf and thigh circumference Trendelenburg's test Thomas's test Schober's test
Neurovascular assessment	Peripheral pulses Full neuroexamination if indicated
To conclude	Examine the joint above and below Thank and cover the patient, and wash your hands

Table 10.7 Generic examination of the musculoskeletal system: a summary

Psychiatry

A psychiatric assessment includes a psychiatric history, Mental State Examination (MSE) and a physical examination. The World Health Organization estimates that mental and neurological disorders are the leading cause of ill health and disability globally. Conditions often remain undiagnosed or improperly treated, which contributes to social isolation and poor functioning.

11.1 Symptoms and signs

Symptoms

Depressive symptoms

Patients may display any of the cognitive and/or biological symptoms listed in the clinical insight box. Depression may also be linked with thoughts of self-harm or suicide, and psychotic symptoms in severe depressive episodes.

Manic symptoms

Mania is characterised by an elevated or irritable mood and can frequently present with psychotic symptoms. The symptoms of mania are: biological (e.g. reduced sleep requirement), cognitive (e.g. lack of insight) and psychotic (e.g. delusions of grandeur). Mania can alternate, sometimes rapidly, with depression. **Hypomania** is a less severe form of mania.

> ## Clinical insight
>
> Diagnosis of depression requires a minimum of 2 weeks of symptoms. The most common core features are:
>
> - **anhedonia**: the inability to gain pleasure from activities that are usually enjoyable
> - **anergia**: lack of energy
> - **depressed mood**: sustained lowering of the mood that responds little to circumstances
>
> Additional biological symptoms include: decreased appetite, sleep disturbance, mood worse in the mornings, loss of libido.
>
> Cognitive symptoms include: loss of confidence or self-esteem, hopelessness, excessive guilt, thoughts of suicide or self-harm, poor concentration.
>
> Psychomotor symptoms include: agitation (speeding up) or retardation (slowing down).

Psychotic symptoms

Psychotic symptoms can occur in a range of neurological, drug-induced and psychiatric conditions. Symptoms include:

- perceptual disturbances, e.g. auditory, tactile or visual hallucinations
- thought disorders, e.g. delusions or disorganised thinking
- negative symptoms, e.g. apathy, poor self-care, blunting of emotional responses, poverty of thought and speech
- psychomotor symptoms:
  - catatonia: excessive/decreased motor activity, e.g. rigidity, posturing, stupor
  - echopraxia: repetitively imitating actions of others

Anxiety

Anxiety can occur in severe discrete episodes (**episodic anxiety** or panic attacks) or can be persistent (**generalised anxiety**). Panic attacks are associated with autonomic symptoms, e.g. palpitations, sweating, shaking and difficulty breathing. A **phobia** is a persistent and irrational fear of a specific object, activity or situation that the individual feels compelled to avoid.

Obsessions and compulsions

Obsessions are recurrent, intrusive and distressing thoughts or impulses that occur involuntarily (e.g. fear of contamination). **Compulsions** are mental or physical operations that the patient feels compelled to perform repetitively, to avoid a dreaded event (e.g. repeating a silent mantra or excessive hand washing). They often

Clinical insight

Negative symptoms are common in schizophrenia and represent a deficit of function. Examples of negative symptoms are:

- **apathy**: lack of interest or enthusiasm
- **alogia**: reduced use of words in spontaneous speech
- **blunted affect**: lack of emotional reactivity with little facial expression
- social withdrawal

Negative symptoms can appear before the first acute positive symptoms (e.g. psychosis) and may be confused with another cause (e.g. adolescence). They can be hardest to treat and persist despite improvement in other aspects. This can frequently lead to social exclusion.

occur together in a condition called obsessive–compulsive disorder (OCD).

Delirium

Delirium is the acute onset of fluctuating disturbance of consciousness with altered cognitions, psychomotor disturbances and changes in the sleep–wake cycle. The mnemonic DELIRIUM is useful for identifying a cause:

- **D** – degenerative, drugs
- **E** – epilepsy (post-ictal states), ethanol (intoxication or withdrawal)
- **L** – liver failure, low oxygen (hypoxia)
- **I** – intracranial (injury to the head, subarachnoid haemorrhage, transient ischaemic attack [TIA], cerebrovascular accident [CVA], meningitis, cerebral abscess)
- **R** – rheumatic chorea
- **I** – infections (pneumonia, septicaemia, urinary tract infection [UTI])
- **U** – uraemia
- **M** – metabolic (electrolyte imbalance/hypoglycaemia)

11.2 The psychiatric assessment

It is of the utmost importance that the psychiatric consultation be carried out in a respectful and calm manner, with a non-judgemental attitude. Developing a relationship of trust will improve the history gained and encourage the patient to be compliant with the examination.

Open questions and active listening are essential in the psychiatric assessment. A fluid consultation may be required, e.g. asking about general background information first to help put the patient at ease. It is important to remain safe when undertaking a psychiatric assessment. Ideally the features of the room should ensure that the consultation is conducted in a safe environment; always position yourself nearest to the door.

The psychiatric history

Collateral history A collateral history can be very helpful in making a diagnosis. It should be taken from a person who knows the patient well; this may be a family member, carer or teacher. Gain information about what the patient is normally like and whether his or her behaviour and/or thoughts are different to usual. Finding out how long the symptoms have been present, any clear triggers and whether they have been present before, may also help in your risk assessment and management plan. Remember to maintain confidentiality when discussing any sensitive issues.

Presenting complaint

Record the patient's reason for consultation in his or her own words. If the patient has several complaints then record them all and find out which is troubling him or her most. If admitting someone, record whether the presentation is voluntary or under the Mental Health Act (MHA in the UK). Also find out the mode of presentation, e.g. did the patient voluntarily present at the emergency department or was he or she referred to outpatient services?

History of presenting complaint

A modified OPERATES+ mnemonic (**Table 11.1**) can be used to gain more detail about the presenting complaint. A key aspect is to determine how the symptoms are affecting the patient's functioning, e.g. 'Is the patient still able to work?', 'How is it affecting the patient's relationships?', 'Has the patient been in trouble with the police?'.

Past psychiatric history

Enquire about:
- previous episodes of mental illness, including severity, chronicity and recovery between episodes
- previous contact with community mental health services, e.g. involvement with mental health nurse, day services or community treatment order
- length of previous hospitalisations: voluntary or under the MHA (assessment or treatment order)
- previous treatments: medications, psychotherapy, electro-convulsive therapy (ECT)
- previous self-harm or suicide attempts

	Mnemonic	Example questions
O	Onset of complaint	When did the problem start? Did the problem start suddenly or over a period of time?
P	Progress of complaint	Has it always been the same?
E	Exacerbating factors	Is there anything that makes it worse?
R	Relieving factors	Is there anything that makes it better?
A	Associated symptoms	Have you had any other problems (psychiatric and/or physical)?
T	Timing	Is there any time of day that you notice this problem more?
E	Episodes of being symptom free	Have you had this problem before? How often do you feel like this? When did you last feel well?
S	Severity	How are the symptoms affecting your social and occupational functioning?
+	Development	How did the problems develop?
+	Precipitating factors	Were there any events that triggered the symptoms (e.g. bereavements, relationship difficulties)?

Table 11.1 Modified OPERATES mnemonic for psychiatric HPC

Past medical and surgical history

A general medical history should be taken. Ask particularly about a history of thyroid disease, neurological disease (e.g. epilepsy) and recent illness. An obstetric history should be taken from women, including recent childbirth.

Drug history

Ask about:
- current or previous prescription medications for medical conditions
- current or previous prescription medications for psychiatric conditions
- over-the-counter medications

- compliance (this is important to establish but may be hard to ascertain until the patient's trust has been gained), side effects and allergies
- overuse of prescription medications

Family history

Establish whether any family members have a history of psychiatric illness because such illnesses often run in families and may inform prognosis.

Social history

The social history is very important in the psychiatric assessment. Enquire about:
- accommodation and with whom the patient lives
- employment and financial situation
- relationships with family members, social network and any dependants; gain a good understanding of the quality of relationships and impact on patient's mental health
- children: find out whether they are safe and who is looking after them
- alcohol and substance misuse (e.g. CAGE questionnaire, page 12):
  - age of onset
  - impact of substance misuse on symptoms
  - previous detox, treatment given or periods of abstinence
- current or previous tobacco use
- religion

Personal history

The personal history (**Table 11.2**) will cover many events of the patient's life from childhood. A premorbid history can be difficult to obtain and collateral history is useful here.

Psychiatric systems review

Patients may not be forthcoming in revealing aspects of their history. They may therefore require prompting about the following:
- anxiety
- bereavement
- delusions

- dementia and/or delirium
- eating disorders
- elevated mood or increased energy

Area of personal history	Questions to ask
Birth and childhood development	*Pregnancy and birth:* 'Were there any known complications?' *Development:* 'Did you attain all your developmental milestones at the appropriate time?'
Growing up	*Childhood:* 'Was it happy?' *Family:* ask the patient to describe all relationships in detail *Trauma:* 'Was there any abuse or significant life event, e.g. divorce of parents?'
School	*Academic performance:* 'What qualifications were obtained?' *Further education:* 'Any undertaken?' *Bullying:* 'Was the patient bullied or did he or she bully others?' *Conduct disorders:* 'Any history of truancy, expulsions or fights?'
Occupational history	*Work record:* ask about jobs held (past and current) and work performance
Relationships	*Partners:* record details on partners both past and present *Dependants:* record list of dependants and quality of relationship with them *Sexual relationships:* if appropriate, ask about sexual relationships, sexual orientation and any history of physical or sexual abuse
Forensic	*Convictions:* ask for details on convictions and any time in prison. Ask if there is any relation to their symptoms
Religious orientation	How important is religion to the patient?
Pre-morbid personality	How would the patient, and others, describe themselves when they are well? (Try to get an idea of how they would get on with people and deal with stress, etc.)

Table 11.2 Personal history

- hallucinations
- impulsivity
- low mood
- obsessions and compulsions
- phobias
- psychotic episodes

Mental State Examination

The aim of the MSE is to provide an objective assessment of the patient's mental functioning at a set point in time. It is the equivalent of a physician's physical examination. The MSE can vary at different points in time and is used to monitor treatment. The MSE begins as soon as the consultation starts. Key information will be gathered during the whole of the consultation and only a few questions may need to be asked at the end of the consultation to complete the MSE.

Appearance and behaviour

How does the patient appear?
- Appropriately dressed?
- Physically fit?
- Age-appropriately dress?
- Evidence of self-harm or neglect?
- Somnolent (sleepy) or hyperalert?

How does the patient behave?
- Does he or she make eye contact?
- What is the quality of the rapport?
- Is there psychomotor agitation?
- Is there evidence of bradykinesia, motor retardation or tremor?

Speech

From the start of the consultation note the rate, quality, flow and volume of the patient's speech, e.g. the patient may have slow, quiet speech with pauses in depression and pressure of speech in mania.

Speech abnormalities can indicate a neurological abnormality (**Table 8.6**). Use the tests described in the Mini-Mental State Examination (MMSE) to test language (**Table 8.8**).

Thoughts

Thought content:

- **Delusions** – a fixed, false belief not accepted by other members of the patient's culture
- **Overvalued ideas** – a preoccupation with a belief that is comprehensible to others
- **Rumination** – repetitive internal debate that is often anxious in nature
- **Disorganised thinking** – common in psychotic patients and can make history taking extremely difficult; these abnormal thought patterns are evident in the disorganised speech

Mood and affect

Mood is a patient's emotional state over a period of time. The patient's subjective mood can be elicited on direct questioning, e.g. 'How have you been feeling in yourself lately?', and should be described in his or her own words. Objectively the patient's mood may be normal (euthymic), elated, low (depressed), anxious, irritable or apathetic.

Describe the patient's **affect**: this is an objective impression of the patient's predominant emotional state at that moment in time. It is assessed by observing posture, emotional reactivity, facial expression and speech. There are two factors to consider here:

1. Congruency: does the affect correspond with the patient's subjectively reported mood?
2. Range of affect: is it normal (reactive), blunted (limited facial expressions or monotonous voice), flat (very little or no expression) or labile (unpredictable changes between extremes of mood)?

Perception

Abnormal perceptions can include the following:

- **Hallucinations:** subjectively experienced sensations in the absence of an appropriate stimulus which can be auditory, visual, gustatory (taste), somatic or olfactory
- **Illusions:** a misperception of a real external stimulus

- **Pseudohallucinations**: a perceptual experience arising from the subjective inner space of the mind, e.g. flashback or internal negative voice

With auditory hallucinations it is important to define if they are heard in the:

- first person (e.g. audible thought or thought echo)
- second person (e.g. critical or command hallucinations speaking to the patient)
- third person (e.g. voices discussing the patient or voices speaking in a 'running commentary')

Insight

Insight is the extent to which the patient understands his or her symptoms being related to a mental illness and whether he or she recognises the need for treatment. It is the strongest predictor for recovery in most severe mental illnesses and may be amenable to psychoeducation.

Cognition

See 'Higher mental function' (below).

Risk assessment

It is essential to undertake an assessment of the patient's risk towards themselves and others. Harm to themselves may include self-harm, suicide or self-neglect. Harm towards others may be physical, sexual or harassment. Risk of harm towards children, either direct or by neglect, must also be specifically assessed. It is common for each to be rated as low, moderate or high. If they are being admitted to hospital, consider compliance with medications, absconding and damage to property.

Suicidal assessment When asking a patient about his or her suicide risk, phrase it in a gentle and tactful way, e.g. 'Many people in your situation have thoughts about harming themselves or even ending their lives; have you ever had thoughts like that?' If yes: 'Have you ever thought of acting on these thoughts?'. Suicidal risk is higher in certain groups. Risks for suicidal ideation can be assessed using the mnemonic SAD PERSONS:

- S – sex (females more likely to attempt, men more likely to succeed)
- A – age (young or old)
- D – depression
- P – previous attempts
- E – ethanol (alcohol) abuse
- R – rational thinking loss
- S – social support lacking
- O – organised plan for suicide
- N – no spouse
- S – sickness, terminal illness?

11.3 Higher mental function

As part of your assessment, perform a brief cognition test such as the Abbreviated Mental Test (AMT) (Table 8.7). If appropriate, subsequently perform a thorough assessment of higher mental function (Table 8.8).

Clinical insight

Physical disease is more prevalent in patients with psychiatric disease than in the general population. Mental health workers should therefore maintain skills in physical examination to ensure that physical illness is diagnosed and treated quickly and appropriately.

Physical examination

A general physical examination should be performed in all patients, with particular attention to the neurological and endocrine systems. This may identify an underlying physical cause of the symptoms (e.g. thyrotoxicosis, encephalitis, HIV infection) or side effects of medications.

11.4 Common investigations

At initial presentation appropriate investigation is required to exclude the possibility of a physical cause. For example, cerebral tumour, stroke, head injury, epilepsy, multiple sclerosis and Parkinson's disease can present with personality change, cognitive deficits and mood change. Endocrine disease, HIV and many other chronic diseases can also present with psychiatric components. Investigations may be required to differentiate delirium from dementia (see page 191).

Consider the following:

- **Blood tests:** full blood count (assessing for anaemia), calcium, thyroid function, renal function, liver function, vitamin B12, folate, glucose
- **Urine tests:** (dipstick, microscopy, culture and sensitivity) for signs of urinary infection, renal or diabetic disease
- **ECG**
- **Head:** CT/MRI

11.5 System summary

A summary of the psychiatric assessment is given in **Table 11.3**.

Preparation	Wash hands; ensure privacy; introduce self and explain examination Gain consent for examination; offer a chaperone
Psychiatric history	Presenting complaint History of presenting complaint Past medical and surgical history Past psychiatric history Drug history Family and social history Personal history Premorbid personality Psychiatric systems review
Mental State Examination	Appearance and behaviour Speech Mood Thought form and content Perceptions Cognitive functioning Insight
Physical examination	Full physical examination if significant symptoms Vital signs Weight

Table 11.3 Psychiatric assessment: a summary

Endocrine system

The endocrine system is a made up of the hypothalamus, pituitary, thyroid, parathyroids, adrenals, pancreas, pineal gland and gonads. The symptoms and signs are diverse and pathologies involving the endocrine system (e.g. diabetes) have huge global health implications.

12.1 System overview

Anatomy review
The thyroid gland

The lobes of the thyroid gland (**Figure 12.1**) curve around the trachea and oesophagus and are partially obstructed by the sternocleidomastoid muscles. The thyroid is attached to the pre-tracheal fascia and therefore moves upwards on swallowing.

Physiology review
The hypothalamopituitary axis

The hypothalamopituitary axis (HPA) is a complex system of homeostatic feedback loops, as summarised in **Figure 12.2**. The hypothalamus, located at the base of the brain, can be thought of as the 'control centre' of the endocrine system. The HPA is the location whereby the neurological and endocrine systems meet to provide homeostatic processes.

Thyroid regulation The hypothalamus produces the thyroid-stimulating hormone (TSH) to stimulate the production of thyroxine (T_4) and triiodothyronine (T_3) (**Figure 12.2**). T_3 is the most active of these two hormones and can act on almost all the cells of the body. It mainly controls metabolism, growth and catecholamine sensitivity.

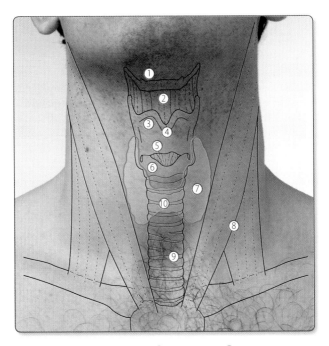

Figure 12.1 Anatomy of the thyroid ①, Body of hyoid; ②, thyrohyoid membrane; ③, thyroid cartilage lamina; ④, laryngeal prominence; ⑤, cricothyroid membrane; ⑥, cricoid cartilage; ⑦, left lateral lobe of thyroid; ⑧, sternocleidomastoid; ⑨, trachea; ⑩, thyroid isthmus.

Glycaemic control

Glycaemic control is reliant on the α and β cells of the pancreas, which secrete glucagon and insulin respectively (**Figure 12.3**). Insulin secretion and resistance are disordered in type 1 and 2 diabetes respectively.

12.2 Symptoms and signs

Endocrine history

Take a full history (**Table 12.1**) using the mnemonic OPERATES+ (Table 1.2) for each presenting complaint or problem.

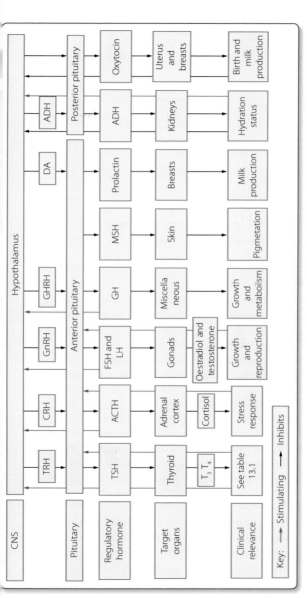

Figure 12.2 Hypothalamopituitary axis: thyroid-releasing hormone (TRH), corticotrophin-releasing hormone (CRH), gonadotrophin-releasing hormone (GnRH), growth hormone-releasing hormone (GHRH), dopamine (DA), thyroid-stimulating hormone (TSH), adrenocorticotrophic hormone (ACTH), follicle-stimulating hormone (FSH), luteinising hormone (LH), growth hormone (GH), melanocyte-simulating hormone (MSH), antidiuretic hormone (ADH); thyroxine (T4); triiodothyronine (T3).

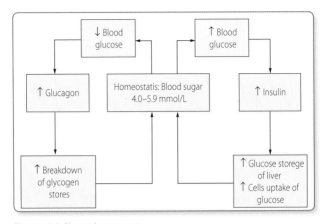

Figure 12.3 Glucose homeostasis.

Symptoms

The endocrine system is complex and affects every body system. Key symptoms are shown here; however, a comprehensive systematic review (Table 1.6) is required. Tiredness is a subjective and common symptom and may be significant if this is a new problem for the patient. Temperature intolerance can present with either excessive or reduced need for clothing.

Polydipsia and polyuria

Polydipsia is excessive thirst. This can be voluntary (psychogenic polydipsia). A good differentiator is whether the patient is waking in the night to drink fluid and pass urine. **Polyuria** is excessive urine production. These are often the first symptoms of diabetes mellitus, diabetes insipidus and hypercalcaemia.

Weight change

This may present as unplanned or unwanted weight gain or loss. Many patients will not know how much weight they have lost, but notice that clothing no longer fits properly. Weight change may be associated with a change in appetite. Endocrine causes of weight loss include hyperthyroidism, diabetes and adrenal

History component	Key points
Presenting complaint	Polydipsia or polyuria Temperature intolerance (hot or cold) Weight change Excessive sweating Skin and hair changes Bowel disturbance Mood changes Lethargy Tremor Palpitations Neck swelling Gynaecomastia or galactorrhoea Visual field disturbance Menstrual irregularities Erectile dysfunction
Past medical history	Thyroid disease or surgery
Drug history	Steroids, contraception, hormone replacement therapy, thyroid replacement
Family history	Autoimmune disorders, diabetes and/or thyroid disease.
Social history	Current or previous tobacco use (quantify it in pack-years)

Table 12.1 The endocrine history

insufficiency. Endocrine causes of weight gain include hypothyroidism, Cushing's disease and polycystic ovary syndrome.

Skin and hair changes

Skin and hair changes are common in endocrine disease. Increased perspiration (sweating) can be seen in hyperthyroidism and hypoglycaemia. Ask about changes in skin pigmentation. In Addison's disease there is generalised increased skin pigmentation (resembling tanned areas), most commonly in light-exposed areas such as the elbows, knees and palmar creases. Hypopigmented patches can be seen in autoimmune-associated endocrine diseases.

Hyperglycaemia and hypoglycaemia

Deranged glycaemic control can be a hallmark of endocrine disease and often presents with non-specific symptoms and signs.

Hyperglycaemia This presents with symptoms of polydipsia, polyuria, weight loss, blurred vision, fatigue or lethargy, seizures and coma. There are usually no signs unless the patient is acidotic (i.e. tachypnoea, acidotic breathing, confusion, dehydration or shock).

Hypoglycaemia This presents with symptoms and signs of anxiety or arousal, palpitations, tremor, sweating, hunger, paraesthesia, cognitive impairment, behavioural changes, seizures, coma, pallor, sweating, tachycardia and/or mildly raised blood pressure (BP).

Signs

Key endocrine signs are shown in **Table 12.2**. Palpitations, gynaecomastia and tremor are described in Chapters 3, 5 and 8 respectively.

General	Mental state: agitation or depression	Change in energy level
Skin	Vitiligo Hirsuitism	Hair loss
Eyes	Exophthalmos Ophthalmoplegia	Visual field defects
Hands	Skin-crease pigmentation Acromegaly Tremor	Carpal tunnel syndrome Palmar erythema
Face	Moon face Coarse face	Pallor
Neck	Goitre	
Breast	Gynaecomastia	Galactorrhoea
Genitalia	Virilisation Pubertal development	Testicular volume
Peripheries	Proximal myopathy Myxoedema	Necrobiosis lipoidica Abnormal reflexes

Figure 12.2 Key signs on endocrine examination

Neck swelling

A **goitre** is an enlargement or swelling of the thyroid gland. Any lumps, bumps and/or swellings should be described (Table 2.7). Differential diagnoses include lymphadenopathy, cysts, lipomas and abscesses.

Visual field disturbance

Tumours (also known as space-occupying lesions) of the pituitary can cause pressure on the optic chiasma, resulting in a bitemporal hemianopia (Figure 9.1).

12.3 Examination of the thyroid

Start with an assessment of the patient's height and weight. Calculate the body mass index (BMI).

Vital signs

See Table 2.2.

Inspection

General Inspection

Expose the neck and upper thorax as a minimum. Inspect for general features of thyroid disease (**Table 12.3**).

Skin, hair and nails

Inspect the skin for colour, dryness, flushing, dermatitis, striae and/or pigmentary changes. Note the quality of hair growth and its distribution. **Thyroid acropachy** is the clubbing and digital swelling associated with Graves' disease.

Limbs

Inspect for a resting tremor and pretibial myxoedema. To assess for a tremor, ask the patient to extend both arms in front with the hands prone. He or she should maintain this for a few seconds. To detect a fine tremor it can be helpful to place a sheet of paper on the hands.

Proximal myopathy

Proximal myopathy manifests as difficulty standing from a

	Hyperthyroid	Hypothyroid
General inspection	Sweaty, flushed, restless	Thin dry hair
Temperature	Warm	Cold
Weight	Underweight	Overweight
Face	Proptosis causing lid retraction Lid lag	Coarse facial features, periorbital skin oedema Malar flush Loss of outer third of eyebrow
Hands	Palmar erythema, tremor and warm sweaty palms	Cold and dry
Pulse	Bounding, tachycardic, irregular (atrial fibrillation)	Bradycardic
Other	Brisk tendon reflexes, goitre	Delayed relaxation of ankle reflex, hoarse voice, goitre

Table 12.3 Thyroid status

sitting position without the patient using their hands. Proximal myopathy can be a sign of hypothyroidism.

The eyes
The eyes should be examined for proptosis and/or lid lag (Chapter 8).

The neck
Inspect the neck from the front and side of the patient for masses, goitres and/or scars. Give the patient a glass of water and ask him or her to take a sip and swallow. As he or she swallows, the thyroid gland should be seen rising.

Palpation
1. Position yourself behind the patient and explain that you will be palpating the neck
2. Encircle the neck with your hands (**Figure 12.4**)

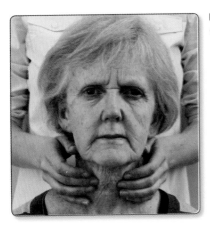

Figure 12.4 Examination of the thyroid.

3. Find the cricoid cartilage using your index and middle finger. The cricoid cartilage is inferior to the laryngeal prominence of the thyroid cartilage (**Figure 12.1**). Alternatively, you may choose to start with your fingers in the midline of the sternal notch, working your way up. The cricoid is the first hard ring that is palpable

4. Palpate immediately inferior to the cricoid for the isthmus of the thyroid

5. Work your way laterally to palpate the lateral lobes of the thyroid. Note the size, consistency (soft or firm) of the thyroid and whether there are any irregularities (including nodules). Is the thyroid fixed or mobile? If it is enlarged, is it nodular or diffusely enlarged? In general, the anterior surface of the lateral lobe should not be larger than the terminal phalanx of the patient's thumb. The right lobe is commonly slightly larger than the left lobe and this asymmetry can be accentuated by a goitre

6. While palpating the thyroid, ask the patient to swallow a sip of water. The thyroid should move upwards on swallowing

7. Palpate for cervical and axillary lymphadenopathy and/or masses (Chapter 2)

Auscultation

Auscultate over the thyroid gland for bruits, indicating increased blood flow.

Tendon reflexes

Assess the tendon reflexes of the ankles. These are brisk in hyperthyroidism and delayed in hypothyroidism.

12.4 Diabetes

Approximately 350 million people worldwide have diabetes, with 3.5 million deaths annually; the rate is predicted to increase by two-thirds by 2030. Eighty per cent of diabetes-related deaths occur in low- or middle-income countries. Type 2 diabetes accounts for 90% of people with diabetes and is largely the result of physical inactivity and excess body weight.

Diabetes review

Diabetes care is now routinely managed in primary care clinics, with the history and examination focusing on diabetes-specific complications

Diabetes history

- Date of diagnosis and mode of presentation
- Form of diabetes (type 1 or 2)
- Current effect of diabetes on quality of life
- Blood sugar monitoring: frequency of monitoring, values and trends, hypoglycaemia or hyperglycaemic episodes (any symptoms noted during these), any significant hypoglycaemic episodes requiring assistance from a third person
- Previous hospitalisations (including diabetic ketoacidosis and hyperosmolar hyperglycaemic non-ketotic coma [HONK])
- Macrovascular complications (e.g. myocardial infarction [MI]) or microvascular complications (e.g. retinopathy)

- Do they attend a retinopathy screening programme or see a podiatrist or dietitian?
- Assessment of cardiovascular risk factors (page 60)
- Any surgery, e.g. amputation, angioplasty, bypass

Diabetes treatment

- Initial management (and its effect)
- Current management (and its effect): oral hypoglycaemics, insulin (type, units, timing), antihypertensives, aspirin, statins, other medications
- Compliance

Social history

- Smoking (pack-year history) and attempts to stop
- Alcohol consumption (units/week)
- Diet (quantity and quality) and its effect on blood sugar control
- Driving status
- Contraception and plans for pregnancy (in women)
- Sexual functioning (in men)

Examination

- Vital signs
- Cardiovascular, respiratory and abdominal examination
- Injection sites (inspect and palpate)
- Signs of autoimmune disease (goitre, vitiligo)
- Feet and peripheries: colour, temperature, capillary refill, pedal pulses, infections, injuries, sensation
- Footwear
- Skin
- Ophthalmology: fundoscopy, cataracts, visual acuity
- Calculate BMI

Investigations

- Blood tests: long-term blood glucose control (HbA1c – glycated haemoglobin), kidney function (urea, creatinine and electrolytes), lipid levels, TSH
- Urine tests: kidney function (albumin:creatinine ratio)

12.5 Common investigations

Common investigations differ depending on the suspected disorder and gland. For example, along with thyroid function tests, ECG or fine-needle biopsy may be indicated in suspected thyroid disease. Investigations may include:

- **Blood and urine concentrations of hormones:** along with measures of the hormones that stimulate/inhibit hormone production [e.g. low blood testosterone confirms hypogonadism; luteinising hormone and follicle-stimulating hormone levels distinguish between primary (testicular) and secondary (e.g. hypothalamic) causes]
- **Dynamic tests:** (provoking a gland to respond): to diagnose diseases not detectable by basal level measurements, e.g. the Synacthen test using synthetic adrenocorticotropic hormone to test adrenal function
- **Imaging:** to visualise structural abnormalities, e.g. ultrasonography to assess thyroid lesions or functional positron emission tomography and scintigraphy to show raised metabolic activity due to tumours

In diabetes, capillary blood glucose monitoring is a cheap and easy test that can be performed in the office for monitoring (normally 4.0–5.9 mmol/L in adults). However, diagnosis requires investigation of plasma glucose levels or HbA1c (glucose bound to haemoglobin, reflecting blood glucose over several weeks).

12.6 System summary

A summary of the thyroid examination is given in **Table 12.4**.

Preparation	Wash hands; ensure privacy; introduce self and explain examination Gain consent for examination; offer a chaperone; position patient (upright) and expose the neck
Vital signs	Temperature; pulse rate and rhythm; respiratory rate; blood pressure
Inspection	General status of the patient (sweating, clothing, skin, hair, weight) Hands; tremor; face; eyes (from front, behind and above the patient); legs Neck (from front and sides); neck as patient swallows a sip of water
Palpation	Identify cricoid; lobes of thyroid; isthmus of thyroid Palpate while patient swallowing water Regional lymph nodes
Auscultation	Auscultate over thyroid
Finish	Deep tendon reflexes Ask patient to stand from seated position Body mass index Thank and cover the patient, and wash your hands

Table 12.4 Examination of the thyroid: a summary

Paediatrics

Paediatrics is the field of medicine for individuals from birth through to the end of adolescence or early adulthood. The human body goes through a huge transition in this period and the pathologies that affect the different age groups vary considerably. Although children are not 'little adults', the systematic approaches to history taking and examination are very similar. Please refer to the relevant system chapters in this book on key concepts of inspection, palpation, etc.

Age definitions
- **Neonate**: first month (28 days)
- **Infant**: 1–23 months
- **Pre-school child**: 2–5 years
- **Child**: 6–12 years
- **Adolescent**: 13–18 years

The clinical environment
The clinical environment is important in paediatric medicine. This should be child friendly in order to put the child and family at ease. The history can be taken as the child is either sat on a carer's knee or playing. Try to establish a good rapport with the caregiver and child. Use this time to carefully observe the child.

13.1 Overview

Children are smaller than adults, yet their anatomy and physiology remain much the same except for some key differences: weight, anatomy (size and shape), physiology (cardiovascular, respiratory and immune function) and psychology (development, intellectual ability and emotional responses).

Anatomy review
Weight
This is very important because drugs and fluids are given based on calculations from weight. Children should be weighed and have their height taken at most consultations and these values plotted on an age-appropriate growth chart. In an emergency it may be appropriate to use a predicted weight, based on age:

- 0–12 months: weight (in kg) = (0.5 × age in months) + 4
- 1–5 years: weight (in kg) = (2 × age in years) + 8
- 6–12 years: weight (in kg) = (3 × age in years) + 7

Body surface area
Younger children have a higher body surface area to weight ratio, making them more prone to hypothermia. Surface area can be calculated for the administration of certain drugs (page 39).

Physiology review
Breathing
An infant has three times, and a 6 year old has double, the minute volume (per kilogram) of an adult. At birth, an infant has approximately 10 million alveoli compared with 300 million by the age of 8 years. Infants rely mainly on diaphragmatic breathing and are therefore more prone to respiratory distress.

Circulation
The circulating volume (per kilogram) is higher in infants (100 mL/kg) compared with children (70–80 mL/kg) and adults (70 mL/kg). They are therefore prone to the effects of blood loss. In infants, stroke volume is small (1.5 mL/kg at birth) but the cardiac index is the highest at any point in life (300 mL/kg per min). These values increase and decrease respectively with age and these changes account for age-dependent heart rates. Systolic blood pressure is age, gender and height dependent (see below).

13.2 Symptoms and signs

The paediatric consultation is significantly more complex in that it is usually triadic, i.e. taken from a third person (caregiver). Take a full history (**Table 13.1**) using the mnemonic OPERATES+ (Table 1.2) for each presenting complaint or problem.

Perinatal history

In neonates and infants a great deal of the history revolves around the maternal perinatal history:

- **Maternal history**: age, blood type, chronic maternal illness (e.g. diabetes), sexually transmitted infections or STIs (herpes, HIV/AIDS), acute or recent illnesses
- **Current pregnancy** (i.e. of infant in question): probable gestational age (last menstrual period [LMP]), prenatal care received, problems with current pregnancy (e.g. pre-eclampsia, bleeding, trauma, infection, surgery, early labour)
- **Drug history during pregnancy**: medications during pregnancy; drug, alcohol, or tobacco use during pregnancy
- **Previous pregnancy and outcomes**: abortions or fetal demise, neonatal deaths, prematurity or postmaturity, jaundice, birth malformations
- **Labour and delivery**: place of birth, presentation (cephalic, breech or transverse), onset and duration of labour, method of delivery, rupture of membranes (prolonged if >18 h), maternal fever during labour, birth weight (plot this with current weight), admission to special care baby unit (SCBU)

Red flags

Paediatric red flags (**Table 13.2**) are signs of, or can suggest, significant illness in children.

> ### Clinical insight
>
> Consultations with adolescents are difficult. Always start by taking the history from the patient first and gaining any additional information from the parents later. Having a short period of time without the parents present may improve the chances of disclosure related to lifestyle. HEADSSS is a useful mnemonic to use for social history: **h**ome, **e**ducation, **e**ating, **a**ctivities, **d**rugs, **s**ex, **s**uicidality, **s**afety.

History component	Key points
Presenting complaint	Shortness of breath Cough Wheeze Stridor Abdominal pain Vomiting Diarrhoea Fits, faints and funny turns Headache Weakness Abnormal gait Hypotonia Cyanosis Heart failure (shortness of breath, poor feeding) Acute limp
Past medical history	Hospital admission, injuries, recurrent or recent infections Perinatal history in infants
Past surgical history	Previous surgery
Development	See **Table 13.3**
Nutrition	Breastfed infants: pattern (frequency, length, etc.), problems with breastfeeding, supplements used Formula-fed infants: pattern (frequency, length, etc.), type of formula used For older infants and children: age of weaning, current dietary intake, number of daily feeds
Drug history	Medications Immunisation history (in children or when clinically relevant) Allergies
Family history	Consanguinity Recurrent miscarriages FH of congenital malformations and/or neonatal death Plot FH (Figure 1.1)
Social history	Parental age, educational level and occupation Current housing Recent travel Parental tobacco, alcohol or illicit drug use Adolescents: use of tobacco, alcohol, illicit drugs and sexual activity

Table 13.1 The paediatric history

Age	Infant <3 months
Airway	Significant stridor Any respiratory sign associated with decreased level of activity
Breathing	Grunting Tachypnoea (respiratory rate >60/min) Moderate or severe respiratory distress
Circulation	Reduced skin turgor Pale, mottled, ashen or blue Cold peripheries Prolonged capillary refill time Unable to rouse or if roused does not stay awake Weak, high-pitched or continuous cry Anuria Haemorrhage Bradycardia or hypotension
Disability	No response to social cues Bulging fontanelle Neck stiffness Status epilepticus Focal neurological signs or focal seizures
Exposure	Temperature ≥38°C (0–3 months) or ≥39°C (3–6 months) Non-blanching rash Bile-stained vomiting

Table 13.2 Paediatric red flags

Such children should be seen, assessed, investigated and treated promptly.

Paediatric extras

The structure of the history remains unchanged from that in adult medicine with an increased emphasis on immunisation, and family and social histories. There are also the following additional areas to cover:

- perinatal history
- developmental milestones (infants and pre-school children)
- nutrition including feeding methods
- detailed immunisation history
- detailed family history, including consanguinity (**consanguinity** is the term referring to parents who are themselves blood relatives)

Key paediatric symptoms

Some system-specific presenting complaints and diagnoses are shown in **Table 13.3**.

Fever

Fever is one of the most common presenting complaints in children. It is usually acute in onset. The history and examination will often reveal a clear diagnosis.

Key paediatric signs

Most clinical signs found in adults can be found in children.

Cardiovascular	Congenital heart disease (e.g. ventricular septal defect [VSD]) Arrhythmias
Respiratory	Viral upper respiratory tract infections (URTIs) Pneumonia Acute asthma Chronic cough Croup
Gastrointestinal	Gastroenteritis Constipation Urinary tract infection Gastro-oesophageal reflux disease (GORD) Cow's milk protein intolerance or allergy
Neurology	Febrile seizure Epilepsy Migraine Cerebral palsy
Musculoskeletal	Transient synovitis Reactive arthritis Septic arthritis Osteomyelitis Perthes' disease Slipped upper femoral epiphysis (SUFE) Juvenile idiopathic arthritis

Table 13.3 Common system-specific paediatric diagnoses

Respiratory distress

Pneumonia remains the biggest killer of children aged <5, globally. Infants and children frequently present with respiratory distress. They are prone to respiratory distress because the chest wall is more pliable and the respiratory muscles are immature. The signs of respiratory distress are:

- **vital signs**: tachypnoea, tachycardia, hypotension
- **airway**: stridor, grunting
- **general**: cyanosis, pallor, decreased level of consciousness, difficulty speaking
- **head and neck**: tracheal tug, nasal flare, head bobbing,
- **chest**: retractions (subcostal, intercostal, supraclavicular), reduced air entry
- **abdomen**: abdominal paradoxical movement

Dehydration

Gastroenteritis is the second biggest killer of children worldwide. Spotting the signs of dehydration (Table 2.4) is crucial in recognising which children need rapid, active rehydration.

Murmurs in children

The classification (Figure 3.9) of murmurs in children is the same as in adults. Auscultate the same four positions as for adults (Figure 3.2). In infants with bounding femoral pulses, palpate and auscultate the left infraclavicular region for the thrill and harsh continuous murmur of **patent ductus arteriosus** (PDA).

In children it is often tempting to auscultate at the start of the examination, when the child is settled. You must not forget to go back and thoroughly complete the full examination in order to gain a diagnosis.

Structurally normal hearts, without pathology, can produce innocent murmurs. The 'Ss' of an innocent murmur are as follows:

- Soft
- Short
- Symptom-free

Clinical insight

It is relatively common to hear a murmur when a child is febrile. Provided that there are no signs of cardiac disease, re-examine the child after the infective period. In most cases the murmur will have disappeared.

- Systolic
- Site – heard over small area
- Sitting and standing – murmur changes with changes of position (decreases in intensity when patient stands)
- Signs – none present
- Special tests – radiograph, ECG normal

13.3 Examining a child

Children need to be examined thoroughly just as you would an adult, although there are some hints and tips for succeeding in this. Your examination should be focused, guided by your history taking.

Hints and tips for paediatric examination

1. **Play**: incorporate play into the consultation; get down to the child's level
2. **Language**: use words children understand (e.g. 'tummy' rather than 'abdomen')
3. **Be opportunistic**: undertake important tasks first while the child is quiet and settled (e.g. auscultating the chest and heart); you may need to start by auscultating or palpating through clothing (but this is bad practice). If the child then becomes unsettled on being undressed you at least have some basic information; if the child remains settled you should re-examine for more accurate signs; if the child is asleep, do not wake him or her. Much of the examination can be performed before the child wakes
4. **Positioning**: do not move a child who is sat comfortably on a carer's knee; the supine position (for abdominal palpation) is threatening to some children, so do this towards the end of the examination
5. **Undressing**: let the carers undress the child
6. **Observation skills**: your examination starts immediately; observe the child in the time you are taking the history
7. **Ear, nose and throat (ENT)**: this is unpleasant for children and should be left until last

Recognising the sick child
Airway, breathing, circulation (ABC)

Your examination begins immediately at the start of the consultation. Make a rapid assessment of the child's ABC (Chapter 15).

Vital signs

The physiology and anatomy of children adapt from birth to late childhood resulting in modified vital sign parameters (**Table 13.4**).

> ## Clinical insight
>
> Tachypnoea and fever are highly suggestive of a lower respiratory tract infection (pneumonia). However, children often breathe faster when they are febrile. Treat the fever with an antipyrexial; if the tachypnoea remains once the fever has settled, there is likely to be a respiratory pathology.

Respiratory rate The respiratory rate in children is naturally higher because of their relatively greater metabolic rate and oxygen consumption.

Blood pressure Blood pressure should be interpreted with age-/gender-/height-dependent centile charts. The 50th centile systolic BP can be calculated using the formula:

$$BP = 85 + (\text{age in years} \times 2)$$

Hypotension is a late and pre-terminal sign of circulatory failure.

	Infant	1–2 years	2–5 years	5–12 years	Adolescent
Pulse rate (beats/min))	110–160	100–150	95–140	80–120	60–90
Respiratory rate (/min)	30–40	25–35	25–30	20–25	14–18
Blood pressure – systolic (mmHg)	80–90	85–95	85–100	90–100	100–140
Temperature (define if oral, etc.) (°C)	35–37				36–37.5
Saturation (%)	94–98				

Table 13.4 Normal vital signs in children

Conscious level In young children it is not possible to fully assess the Glasgow Coma Scale (GCS) and so the alert, voice, pain, unresponsive (AVPU) scale should be employed (Table 15.3).

Capillary refill time This is commonly used in paediatric assessment (Chapter 2). A delayed CRT can indicate poor skin perfusion, which is a helpful sign in early septic shock. A normal capillary refill time (CRT) should be ≤2 s. Peripheral CRT can be delayed by shock, dehydration, hypotension, metabolic acidosis and/or hypothermia. A delayed CRT can be caused by hypothermia (or even cold ambient temperature), so a central CRT is more reliable.

System-specific examinations

The system-based examinations, described in Chapters 2–6, remain largely unchanged. However, you may not be able to do it in the strict and systematic order you follow with an adult. There are some system-specific differences in paediatric examination (**Table 13.5**).

Ear, nose and throat

The ENT examination is much the same as described in Chapter 2. Explain clearly to the child and carer what the examination involves. Positioning is the most important part of getting this examination right in children.

To inspect the tympanic membranes, do the following:
- Sit the child on the carer's lap facing sideways
- The head can then be held firmly but comfortably against the carer's chest
- Support the otoscope holding your hand on the child's head, then if the child moves the otoscope moves with him or her
- Turn the child round and repeat with the opposite ear

Throat inspection is difficult and should be carried out as follows:
- Sit the child on the carer's lap, facing forward, with the child's back firmly against the carer's chest and one arm around the child's chest (being sure to encircle both the child's arms to prevent thrashing and injury to the clinician)

	Inspection	Palpation	Percussion and Auscultation
Cardiovascular	JVP and hepatojugular reflex difficult to assess in younger children Scars common in congenital heart disease	In infants, assess pulse at the brachial artery	Non-fixed second heart sound splitting normal Non-pathological murmurs common in acute illness
Respiratory	Respiratory distress	Small thorax cages	Local signs are difficult to interpret or absent
Gastrointestinal	Gastrostomies common in chronic illness	Voluntary guarding common Rectal examination rarely required	
Neurology	Neurocutaneous lesions may be present Gait is important Use AVPU, not GCS	Palpate anterior fontanelle in infants	
Musculoskeletal	pGALS	Perform Ortolani's and Barlow's tests in infants	
AVPU, alert, voice, pain, unresponsive; GCS, Glasgow Coma Scale; JVP, jugular venous pressure; pGALS, paediatric gait, arms, legs, spine.			

Table 13.5 System-specific differences in paediatric examination

- Ask the carer to hold the child's forehead with the other hand and tip it back slightly
- Demonstrate to the child how you would like him or her to open the mouth. You may wish to ask them: 'Show me what you had for breakfast' or 'Roar like a lion'
- Use a tongue depressor to visualise the oropharynx (Figure 2.7)

Growth and nutrition

Growth in children is multifactorial, but grossly dependent on nutrition and thyroid function in the infant years, growth hormone in the childhood years and sex hormones in adolescence. Disorders of these will affect growth, as will chronic illness.

Clinical insight

Many clinicians avoid ENT examination, because it can be distressing for the child, carer and/or clinician. However, unwarranted hospital admission, blood tests and treatments can be avoided, all of which are more distressing in the long term. Occasionally a child needs to be held firmly by a carer to gain a full view of the oropharynx. Warn the carer and child that he or she may gag as you inspect the tonsils.

Plotting on a growth chart

All children should have their height and weight plotted on an age- and sex-appropriate growth chart. An infant who is born prematurely (<37/40) should have his or her growth plotted at a corrected age until 1 year of life. In an emergency a predicted weight may be required.

Malnutrition   Globally, more than a third of under-5 deaths are attributable to malnutrition. **Severe malnutrition** is defined as the presence of severe wasting (<70% weight for height or <−3 standard deviations) and/or oedema. It is therefore diagnosed both clinically and using specially designed growth charts (from the World Health Organization) that compare height against weight. This takes account of **stunting** (reduced height because of chronic poor nutrition). Malnutrition must be treated aggressively because concurrent illness can lead to mortality rates of up to 50%.

Marasmus is caused by inadequate intake of all nutrients (in particular carbohydrate), whereas **kwashiorkor** is caused by inadequate protein intake (**Table 13.6**).

13.4 Development assessment

A basic assessment of development should be undertaken in all pre-school children. Development refers to the acquisition of skills in four domains:

1. gross motor

	Marasmus	**Kwashiorkor**
Clinical features	Emaciated and weak appearance Thin, dry skin Thin, sparse hair Redundant skinfolds	Severe generalised oedema ('moon face') Dry, atrophic, peeling skin Skin hyperpigmentation Dry, dull, hypopigmented hair Hepatomegaly (due to fatty liver infiltrates) Distended abdomen (due to dilated intestinal loops)
Vital signs	Bradycardia Hypotension Hypothermia	Usually normal
Weight and height	Reduced weight and height for age	Normal or nearly normal weight and height for age

Table 13.6 Types of malnutrition

2. fine motor and vision
3. language and hearing
4. social

The developmental assessment should start with a history to identify any parental concerns, behavioural problems (e.g. inattention, impulsivity) and family history of developmental problems. Developmental milestones (**Table 13.7**) are medians and there is normal variation between children.

Developmental delay

Developmental delay is delay in attaining developmental milestones. Delay is defined as performance that is ≥2 standard deviations below the mean for the age of the child, as assessed using standardised testing. Isolated delay is delay in just one of the four domains (e.g. isolated speech delay). Global developmental delay is delay in two or more of the domains.

Common genetic disorders

Inherited disorders commonly first present in childhood (e.g. Down's syndrome) and have therefore often been considered

Age (months)	Gross motor	Fine motor and vision	Language and hearing	Social
3	Raises head to 90° when prone, head control when supine	Fixes and follows through 180°	Turns head to sound, coos	Smiles socially
6	Sits un-supported, rolls front to back	Voluntary grasp of objects, transfers objects between hands	Babbles	Holds bottle when feeding
9	Crawls, pulls to stand	Immature pincer grasp, throws objects	Says mama, dada indiscriminately	Finger feeds, waves bye-bye
12	Cruises between objects, walks	Mature pincher grip, bangs objects together	Uses two words, understands 'no' and name	Stranger awareness, imitates, claps hands
15	Walks stably	Scribbles in imitation, mature pincer grip	Four to six words, follows one-step command	Uses spoon and cup
18	Runs unstably, carries toy while walking	Scribbles spontaneously, turns two to three pages at a time	Seven to ten words, points to named body parts	Copies parent's task (sweeping), plays around other children
24	Walks up and down steps without help, runs stably	Removes shoes, pants, imitates stroke with pencil, turns single pages of a book	50-word vocabulary, two-word sentence, follows two-step command	Parallel play, plays alone

Table 13.7 Developmental milestones

Contd...

Age (months)	Gross motor	Fine motor and vision	Language and hearing	Social
36	Can alternate feet when going up steps	Copies circle, undresses completely, unbuttons	250+ words, three- to four-word sentences	Plays well with others, shares, takes turns
48	Hops, skips	Copies a square, buttons clothing, dresses completely, catches ball	Knows colours, sings songs, asks questions, counts to 10	Plays cooperatively with group of children
60	Alternates feet going down steps	Copies a triangle, writes name	Counts to 20	Chooses own friends, role play

Table 13.7 *Contd...*

the work of paediatric practice. **Syndromes** are recognised collections of clinical features that may or may not have a known genetic cause.

13.5 Examination of the newborn baby

APGAR score

The APGAR score is used to identify newborn babies who may require immediate resuscitation. Five areas are assessed (colour, pulse rate, reflex irritability, tone and breathing), each receiving a score or 0, 1 or 2 (**Table 13.8**). **Reflex irritability** was previously assessed by suctioning the oropharynx or nose, but now it is felt appropriate to stimulate the child with firm rubbing of the sole of the foot. The newborn is 'scored' at 1, 5 and 10 min of age. Scores of ≤3 = critically low (immediate resuscitation required), 4–6 = fairly low (resuscitation may be required), 7–10 = generally normal (no resuscitation required).

APGAR	Name	Score of 0	Score of 1	Score of 2
Colour	Appearance	Blue or white	Peripheral cyanosis Centrally pink	Pink throughout
Pulse rate (beats/min)	Pulse	Absent	<100	>100
Reflex irritability	Grimace	No response to stimulation	Grimace or feeble cry when stimulated	Grimace
Muscle tone	Activity	None or floppy	Some limb flexion	Flexed arms and legs that resist extension
Breathing	Respiration	Absent	Weak, irregular, gasping	Strong, lusty cry

Table 13.8 The APGAR score

The postnatal check

Every baby should have a postnatal check in the first few days of life and this is often referred to as the 'baby check'. It is essentially a screening test and so it is not 100% sensitive or specific and will miss some diagnoses. Start with a perinatal history. Is there any family history of note, in particular disorders of the hips, heart or hearing?

Examination

The newborn baby examination is simply a thorough examination from top to bottom and front to back (**Table 13.9**). Any abnormalities should be discussed with the family and appropriately investigated and/or managed.

Education

The postnatal check is an invaluable opportunity to educate new parents. Give advice about exclusive breastfeeding.

General	Tone Posture Colour	Moro's reflex Dysmorphic appearance
Vital signs	Pulse (100–160 beats/ min) Respiratory rate (<60/min)	Temperature Oxygen saturation (pre- and post-ductal)
Eyes	Red reflexes Movements	Position and size Eye discharge
Head	Shape Anterior fontanelle Suture lines Trauma	Cephalohaematoma Ear shape, positions and/ or tags Head circumference
Nose and mouth	Patent nares Cleft palate Jaw size	Tongue size Sucking reflex Rooting reflex
Neck	Sternocleidomastoid tumour	
Chest	Shape or deformity Clavicles Apex Heart sounds	Breath sounds and added sounds Respiratory effort Breast development or discharge
Abdomen	Shape or distension Hepatosplenomegaly	Kidneys or bladder palpable Umbilicus
Hands	Digits Palmar creases	Palmar grasp
Limbs	Normal limb movements Full range of movements Femoral pulses	Hips (Ortolani's and Barlow's tests) Feet for talipes Stepping reflex

Table 13.9 Examination of the newborn baby

Newborn babies should be placed 'back to sleep' (i.e. in the supine position) until 6 months of age to reduce cot death (sudden infant death syndrome or SIDS) which peaks at 2–4 months.

13.6 Assessment of child mistreatment

It is the responsibility of all professionals (including clinicians) to protect children and young people from mistreatment. Every paediatric consultation is an opportunity to identify children who may be being mistreated and must always be considered.

Mistreatment can come in the form of commission or omission and is classified into four types:

1. physical abuse
2. emotional abuse
3. sexual abuse
4. neglect

If you have any concerns that a child is being mistreated, share your concerns with a senior colleague. Document your concerns in the patient's records. Never keep your concerns to yourself.

Elderly patients

Low fertility rates and longer life expectancy are resulting in a worldwide increase in the proportion of people aged >60 years. This, together with higher rates of disease in this population, mean that being an expert at assessing older patients is a vital role for the general clinician.

14.1 First principles

Chronological versus functional age

Chronological age is an unreliable index of a person's functional capabilities. **Functional age** is a combination of chronological, physical, psychological and emotional age. These can be assessed by age, activities of daily living (ADLs) (Table 1.5). Mini-Mental State Examination (Table 8.8) and psychiatric assessment (Chapter 10) respectively.

Age-associated physiological changes

Ageing (senescence) is the gradual irreversible change in structure and function that occurs as a result of the passage of time. Factors such as gender, genetics, environment and lifestyle will inevitably affect these processes. These physiological changes come with an increased susceptibility to particular diseases:

- **Cardiovascular**: reduced cardiac output, increase in blood pressure, arteriosclerosis and reduced exercise tolerance
- **Respiratory**: reduced vital capacity, forced expiratory volume in 1 second (FEV_1), forced vital capacity (FVC) and peak expiratory flow rate (PEFR), impaired gas exchange and slower expiratory flow rates
- **Gastrointestinal**: reduced motility, atrophic gastritis, slower colonic transit, reduced energy requirements and altered hepatic drug metabolism
- **Nervous system,** including higher senses: hearing loss, reduced visual acuity, muscle mass and/or mental agility or ability

- **Musculoskeletal**: decline in bone mass, reduced muscle mass, degenerative joint changes

14.2 Symptoms and signs

History taking

When taking a history from an older patient (**Table 14.1**) you must always assume that he or she is fully capable of giving a history and autonomous in the ability to understand information and make decisions about him- or herself.

History component	Key points
Presenting complaint	Immobility Instability and/or falls Incontinence Intellectual impairment (e.g. confusion) Iatrogenic illness (e.g. polypharmacy) Impaired senses (hearing and vision) Pressure sores
Past medical history	Often extensive
Past surgical history	The patient may forget past operations or certain conditions so it is important to perform a thorough system review (Table 1.6) Previous surgery
Drug history	All drugs, doses and administrations should be noted Always attempt to see a recent prescription Contacting the family doctor for clarification on details may be required Note polypharmacy Ask about side effects Immunisation history, including seasonal Influenza vaccine.
Family history	Relevant family history
Social history	Smoking and alcohol Social support networks (informal or formal) in place Living arrangements and any home modifications Basic ADLs and instrumental ADLs (Table 1.5)
ADLs, activities of daily living.	

Table 14.1 The history in an elderly patient

There are some simple steps that can be established quickly and early in the consultation which will not only guide the consultation, but also optimise the patient's ability to give a full history:

1. Can the patient see and hear you?
2. Is the patient comfortable and at ease?
3. Is his or her language normal?
4. Is his or her behaviour normal?
5. Is there immediate evidence of support (family, friends or other)?
6. Have you introduced yourself appropriately and does the patient understand your role as a doctor?

The history in an older patient requires patience because it can often be extensive. It is important to minimise interrupting the patient, but try to keep the history focused. Time should also be allowed for a slower pace of the consultation than with a younger adult. It is important to maintain the patient's individual right to autonomy and confidentiality; however, many consultations will require a history from a third party (e.g. a family member).

Older patients often minimise symptoms either because they are worried about 'making a fuss' or because they have coped with the symptom for such a long time. Take each symptom seriously. Never discount a symptom as simply 'part of old age' (e.g. weight loss), but instead make this a diagnosis of exclusion.

> ## Clinical insight
>
> Identify hearing and visual impairment early in the consultation. Sensory impairment can falsely present as neurological disorders and confusion. If a hearing aid is in place, ensure that it is functioning. If you suspect a hearing impairment, examine the ear with an otoscope and request a full audiology assessment. A full vision assessment should be performed, in particular visual acuity (page 214).

> ## Clinical insight
>
> Older patients are much more likely to have multiple presenting complaints. Break the history into a series of problems. These problems may be symptoms, signs, established diagnoses or functional deficits.

Symptoms

The 'geriatric giants' are immobility, instability, incontinence, intellectual impairment and iatrogenic problems.

Clinical insight

Diagnosis in elderly people is not always straightforward. Multiple diagnoses are common so, when examining the patient, take note of seemingly incidental findings. Furthermore, recognise that each symptom or sign may have more than one cause (e.g. breathlessness may be a result of either respiratory or cardiac disease). Finally, remember that the typical pattern of symptoms or signs leading to a diagnosis may not be present (e.g. pneumonia may present simply with confusion). Or, there may be an absence of chest pain in acute coronary syndromes with associated autonomic or diabetic neuropathy).

Immobility

Almost always multifactorial, immobility is a common presenting problem. The timing of immobility can lead to a diagnosis: acute (e.g. delirium, fracture) or chronic (e.g. arthritis, cerebellar disease, dementia).

Instability and/or falls

Older people should be routinely asked whether they have fallen in the past year. If they have fallen, determine the frequency, context and characteristics of the fall(s). If a patient is experiencing significant falls, a full falls assessment should be undertaken:

- **Falls history:** frequency, context, characteristics; injuries sustained; assessment of osteoporosis risk and continence; assessment of continence; medication review; social history; home hazards and adjustments
- **Examination:** nutrition assessment; cardiovascular examination; neurological examination; gait; GALS (page 223) and musculoskeletal examination
- **Senses:** audiology assessment
- **Cognition:** Abbreviated Mental Test (AMT)

Incontinence

Incontinence of urine (page 145) and faeces is more common in elderly people and can be disabling.

Intellectual impairment and confusion

Dementia and delirium are chronic and acute confusional states, respectively.

Dementia This is a form of memory disturbance, with at least one of the following disturbances: aphasia, apraxia, agnosia and/or disturbance in executive functioning. Diagnosis of dementia can be made only after a comprehensive assessment, including history taking, physical examination, cognitive and Mental State Examination (MSE) and a review of medication. A clinical cognitive assessment such as the Mini-Mental State Examination (MMSE) should be used, but further neuropsychological testing may also be required.

Delirium This is a disorder characterised by confusion, inattentiveness, disorientation, delusions, hallucinations and agitation. Causation is varied.

Iatrogenic

The side effects of medications should be considered as potential causes for presenting symptoms and signs. Elderly people are more at risk of these effects because they are often on multiple medications (polypharmacy), metabolise medications differently and can have erratic compliance.

14.3 Examination

The examination starts and continues throughout the consultation. In most respects the examination remains the same as the examinations described in Chapters 2–12; however, it may not be possible to do these in the strict and systematic order, as with a younger, more mobile adult. There are some system-specific differences (see below) in older patients.

Vital signs
Temperature
The baseline temperature in elderly people is lower than in younger adults. The ability to develop fever is also often impaired and elderly patients with severe infections may exhibit only modest temperature rises. Therefore, a temperature of $\geq 37.5°C$ is considered abnormal.

Pulse rate
The stress response of an increased heart rate can be lost in older patients, in particular those on medications such as beta-blockers or those with concurrent autonomic dysfunction.

Bradyarrhythmias and tachyarrhythmias can lead to cardiovascular collapse.

Respiratory rate and oxygen saturation

Respiratory rate should be measured and interpreted as in a younger adult. However, poor peripheral perfusion or cold peripheries can lead falsely to low readings on a pulse oximeter, so oxygen saturation should be interpreted alongside clinical judgement.

Blood pressure

An assessment of blood pressure should include lying and standing (or sitting) measurements (page 32). It is important that any accompanying changes in the heart rate are also noted. If the patient mounts a tachycardia, this indicates that he or she may be hypovolaemic, whereas no associated tachycardia with a drop in blood pressure indicates autonomic dysfunction. Orthostatic (postural) hypotension is a common cause of falls in elderly patients.

Inspection

Nutrition

A full assessment of nutrition should be performed (Chapter 2). Poorly fitting clothes and dentures can give clues to undernutrition. The body mass index (BMI) (page 38) is useful, but take into account loss of height from vertebral disease. Skinfold thickness can be useful in these patients.

Skin

The skin of elderly patients bruises easily (**senile purpura**). Wrinkles are due to ultraviolet light exposure. Other signs of sun damage include basal cell carcinoma, squamous cell carcinoma, malignant melanoma and keratoacanthoma. Do not underestimate the importance of regularly examining pressure areas, these include:

- back of the head and ears
- shoulder
- elbow
- hip

- lower back and buttocks
- greater trochanter
- inner knees
- heel

You should assess whether the skin is intact, frail, erythematous, broken or ulcerated. Always examine the feet and legs. Leg ulcers are more common in older age (caused by venous and/or arterial disease) and are often resistant to healing, particularly in patients with diabetes.

System-specific examinations

In older patients there are some system-specific differences in the examination and/or findings.

Head and face

- **Temporal artery:** palpate for tenderness over the temporal artery (suggesting temporal arteritis)
- **Eyes:** check for eye signs, visual acuity and visual fields (chapter 9)
- **Ears:** perform an audiological assessment (chapter 9)
- **Mouth:** check for ulcers, dental or denture hygiene and voice quality

Cardiovascular

Heart sounds Aortic sclerosis can be heard as a non-radiating systolic murmur in the aortic region. Calcification of the mitral valve can be heard as pansystolic mitral regurgitation.

Peripheral vascular disease This should include: inspection for peripheral skin changes, palpation of the peripheral pulses and for an aortic aneurysm, performing an ankle–brachial pressure index or ABPI (Table 3.9) and auscultating over the carotids for a bruit.

Respiratory

Spine and posture Kyphosis (Figure 10.3) due to vertebral degeneration can reduce respiratory function.

Age-related pulmonary crackles Not all crackles in older patients are pathological. Age-related pulmonary crackles are caused by gas trapping through age-related loss of pulmonary elasticity. The risk of audible crackles increases approximately threefold for every 10 years after the age of 45 years. Be vigilant for other signs of respiratory disease. A chest radiograph is often required to define any lung pathology.

Inhaler technique A poor technique (e.g. due to hand arthritis) could be misinterpreted as a sign of worsening respiratory symptoms.

Gastrointestinal

Abdominal examination This can be limited by poor mobility, kyphosis or orthopnoea. Faecal impaction is common and can have serious consequences (e.g. obstruction).

Rectal examination This is an important part of the assessment of an elderly patient with incontinence, constipation, change in bowel habit and/or iron deficiency anaemia.

Neurological

Communication Problems in communication should be established early in the consultation (Table 8.6).

Screening examination Start with a **screening assessment**, e.g. 'get-up-and-go test' (see below). Follow this with a full neurological examination (Chapter 8) where possible. Each sign needs to be put in the context of the patient's ability to understand the instructions, ability to perform (e.g. reduced power) and any potential pathology.

Gait assessment and gait speed Where possible, a gait assessment should be performed (page 169). Gait speed is a reliable and quick measure of functional ability in older patients. It has well-documented predictive value for disability, cognitive decline, falls, hospitalisation, care home admissions and mortality. Although there are several methods described, the key is to always use the same format with the same patient and document this. Ask the patient to walk at a 'usual pace' from a standing start over a set distance. An expected gait speed is 1.2 m/s.

Musculoskeletal

Get-up-and-go test Similar to gait speed, this is an excellent predictor of functionality and future outcomes. Prepare an appropriate, clear environment. Ask a seated patient to rise (without using hands if possible), walk 3 metres, turn and return to the chair and sit down (again without using hands if possible). You should watch each phase of the test and be ready to support an unsteady patient. Serial timed tests can also be used to monitor response to rehabilitation.

Cognition

The AMT score (Table 8.7) is a quick, standardised method for detecting and monitoring cognition. With sensitivity, explain to the patient that you wish to test his or her memory by asking a few straightforward questions. If it reveals a likely impairment, an MMSE should be performed (Table 8.8).

> ### Clinical insight
>
> If there is a suspicion of cognitive impairment, assess this early in the consultation. Mental functioning reduces with fatigue. A minor illness (e.g. constipation, or urinary tract infection) can have a significant effect on the cognitive function in older patients.

Psychiatric assessment

Do not forget psychiatric illnesses in elderly patients. If your consultation leads to any concern, undertake a full assessment including a MSE (Chapter 10).

> ### Clinical insight
>
> Confounders to a mental test score:
> - level of education
> - cultural background
> - hearing and vision impairment
> - speech disorders
> - depression
> - drugs (e.g. sedatives) and alcohol

What happens next?

Basic dementia screen

Here are a series of tests that should be performed when dementia is suspected:

- Blood tests (FBC [full blood count], U&Es [urea and electrolytes], LFTs [liver function tests], TFTs [thyroid function tests], glucose, calcium, vitamin B_{12} and folate)

- MSU (midstream specimen of urine)
- Chest radiograph, electrocardiogram or electroencephalography as appropriate
- MRI is preferable to CT to aid diagnosis of subtype of dementia

Multidisciplinary team assessment

For an elderly patient with multiple or significant problems, a comprehensive assessment by a multidisciplinary team (MDT) may be required. This comprises: a physician, nurse, social worker, occupational therapist, physiotherapist, dietitian, pharmacist, psychiatrist, audiologist, podiatrist, optician and/or psychologist. The MDT assesses:

- advanced care preferences
- cognition
- dentition
- functional capacity (ADLs and instrumental ADLs [IADLs])
- fall risk
- financial
- living situation
- mood
- nutrition and weight change
- polypharmacy
- sexual function
- social support
- spirituality
- urinary incontinence
- vision and hearing

14.4 System summary

A summary of the examination in an older patient is given in **Table 14.2**.

Preparation	Wash hands; ensure privacy; introduce self and explain examination to patient Gain consent for examination; offer a chaperone, position patient; expose area being examined; examine from the patient's right side
Vital signs	Temperature Pulse rate; respiratory rate; saturation (what is the inspired oxygen?) Blood pressure (lying and standing)
General inspection	Inspection of environment for clues (e.g. oxygen mask, inhalers, sputum pot) General comfort and breathing pattern Nutrition assessment
Head and face	Cranial nerves Temporal artery tenderness
Eyes	General inspection Acuity Assessing fields
Ears	Audiological assessment
Mouth	Dental hygiene Ulcers Voice quality
Neck	Jugular venous pressure Carotid bruits Thyroid examination
Chest	Inspection of chest (scars, symmetry, deformity) Apex beat Auscultation of heart sounds
Pulmonary	Barrel chest; work of breathing Percuss chest (anterior, posterior, axillae, clavicles) Auscultation of lung fields
Breast	Masses; skin changes
Abdomen	Inspection of abdomen; palpation Rectal examination (especially in men)
Neurological	Inspection for tremor; tone; power Reflexes; sensation

Table 14.2 Examination of an elderly patient: a summary

Contd...

Musculoskeletal	GALS assessment; range of movements (active and passive) Full gait assessment including gait speed Joint swelling
Skin	Dermatological disease; foot hygiene and health; ulceration
Peripheries	Peripheral vascular examination ABPI
Finish	Full ear, nose and throat examination Thank and cover the patient and wash your hands
ABPI, ankle–brachial pressure index; GALS, gait, arms, legs, spine.	

Table 14.2 *Contd...*

Critically ill patients

Problems with the airway, breathing or circulation have the capacity to kill or seriously harm a patient very swiftly. In the critically ill patient, the priority of history and management moves from finding an underlying diagnosis to identifying and treating symptoms and/or signs while providing potentially life-saving treatment. An approach to a critically ill patient should be calm, focused and swift. Practising the following, will help assess the patient in a confident and safe manner.

15.1 Primary survey

This ABCDE approach is often referred to as the 'primary survey' (**Table 15.1**). Examination of the patient should be focused and

A – airway	Check airway patency Consider cervical spine injury
B – breathing	Respiratory rate Oxygen saturation Colour Effort of breathing Chest auscultation
C – circulation	Heart rate Pulse volume Blood pressure Auscultation of heart sounds Capillary refill time – in children
D – disability	Glasgow Coma Scale/AVPU Posture Pupils
E – environment/ exposure	Temperature Skin
G – glucose	Check patient's blood glucose
AVPU, alert, voice, pain, unresponsive.	

Table 15.1 Primary survey

targeted, dependent on the emerging situation. If a patient has collapsed, always ensure your own safety when approaching him or her. Check for a response by gently shaking the shoulders and asking loudly 'Are you alright?'.

A – airway

Occlusion of the airway will rapidly lead to death. Without any form of oxygenation, circulatory collapse and irreversible neurological damage will start to occur within minutes. Partial occlusion of the airway will buy more time, but irreversible damage can still occur due to hypoxia. It should always be assumed that a partial occlusion has the potential to progress to full occlusion. Always start high-flow oxygen using a mask with a reservoir bag (page 94), pending further information from oxygen saturation measurements and arterial blood gases.

History

A brief history from bystanders or relatives while making your assessment could lead to a cause and may be life saving, e.g. if there is a history suggestive of an inhaled foreign body or there has been a drug overdose. Ask for the presence of neck pain in patients who have sustained a head injury or multiple trauma.

Examination

It should be immediately obvious if the airway is totally oc-cluded. Initially, the patient will be extremely distressed and will make vigorous attempts to breathe with no success. The patient may point to the throat and his or her appearance may be cyanosed. Within a few minutes, the patient will lose consciousness and chest movements will cease. Immediate in-terventions will be life saving. The signs of a partially obstructed airway are less clear:

- **Abnormal sounds:** stridor and/or gurgling
- **Abnormal chest movements:** 'see-saw' or 'rocking-horse' respiration (paradoxical movement where the chest is drawn in and the abdomen expands on inspiration)
- **General appearance:** agitation, central cyanosis (this is a late sign of airway obstruction)

B – breathing

Normal breathing patterns are reliant on a patent airway. For this reason, the airway assessment must always take precedence. The next priority is to assess and manage any breathing problems.

History

Determine if the breathing problem is acute or chronic. There may be one cause or multifactorial causes (e.g. a patient with chronic lung problems who develops a chest infection after a chest wall injury). If possible, take a brief focused history. The causes of acute respiratory failure are:

- **lung disorders** (e.g. asthma, chronic obstructive pulmonary disease [COPD], pulmonary embolism [PE])
- **lung injury** (e.g. aspiration, contusion)
- **decreased respiratory effort** (e.g. muscle weakness)
- **decreased respiratory drive** (e.g. central nervous system depression)

Examination

Conduct a focused respiratory examination (Chapter 4). Essentials would include: respiratory rate or rhythm, oxygen saturation, inspection for colour and effort of breathing and auscultation of the chest.

Assisting breathing

Target-driven oxygen therapy is the most commonly used emergency treatment for respiratory disorders (page 94). Definitive management will depend on the underlying diagnosis.

C – circulation

The circulatory system needs to be adequately oxygenated to serve any useful purpose. Therefore, do not assess the circulation until airway and breathing issues have been sufficiently managed.

History

Signs and symptoms of cardiac disease may include chest pain, shortness of breath, syncope, dysrhythmias, hypotension, poor peripheral perfusion and an altered mental state. There may or may not be a previous history of cardiac disease.

Causes of acute circulatory problems:

- **Hypovolaemia**: haemorrhage and gastrointestinal loss
- **Cardiogenic:** primary myocardial failure (e.g. ischaemia, arrhythmias, valvular damage, cardiomyopathy) or secondary myocardial failure (e.g. hypoxia, drugs)
- **Obstructive:** pulmonary embolism, tamponade, aortic dissection
- **Distributive:** sepsis or anaphylaxis

The sites of massive haemorrhage are the chest, abdomen, pelvis, long bones, and/or external bleeding

Examination

Conduct a focused cardiovascular examination (Chapter 3) Essentials would include: heart rate, pulse volume and blood pressure.

D – disability

Once the airway, breathing and circulation have been stabilised, attention can turn to the neurological system. Common causes of unconsciousness can be remembered using the mnemonic AEIOU TIPS (**Table 15.2**).

A	Alcohol
E	Epilepsy, electrolyte, endocrine
I	Infection (sepsis, meningitis, encephalitis)
O	Overdose, oxygen deprivation
U	Uraemia
T	Trauma, temperature
I	Insulin
P	Poisoning, psychiatric
S	Stroke, shock

Table 15.2 AEIOU TIPS: mnemonic for causes of reduced consciousness or coma

Examination

Conduct a focused neurological examination (Chapter 8). Essentials would include: an assessment of the Glasgow Coma Scale (GCS) or AVPU (alert, voice, pain, unresponsive) (**Table 15.3**), posture and pupils (Figure 9.7).

Glucose Hypo-/hyperglycaemia is an important cause of impaired consciousness and a bedside glucose test should always be performed.

E – exposure

The final aspect of the primary survey is a brief examination of the rest of the patient

> ### Clinical insight
>
> In general, if a patient is able to engage in a lucid conversation with you, their ABCDE status is not critical at that moment. In order to talk, the patient will have an adequate airway with adequate ventilation. By engaging in normal conversation, the implication is that the brain is perfused with oxygenated blood. Therefore, always start your assessment with an open-ended question (e.g. 'Can you tell me where it is hurting?') and have a higher degree of concern if the patient is unable to answer appropriately.

Score	Eye opening	Verbal response	Motor response	
1	None	None	None	U = unresponsive
2	To pain	Incomprehensible	Extension to pain	V = responds to voice
3	To speech	Inappropriate	Abnormal flexion to pain	
4	Spontaneously	Confused	Flexion or withdrawal to pain	P = responds to pain
5		Oriented	Localises to pain	
6			Obeys commands	A = Alert
AVPU, alert, voice, pain, unresponsive.				

Table 15.3 Glasgow Coma Scale (GCS) with corresponding AVPU scale for children

to identify any signs of an emergency condition (e.g. purpuric rash in meningococcal septicaemia). Thoroughly inspect the skin and assess the patient's temperature.

15.2 Secondary survey

Once the primary survey has been completed and the patient has been stabilised, progress to a secondary survey (**Table 15.4**).

Head and neck	Eyes Ear, nose and throat Cranial nerves Fundoscopy Tracheal position Carotid arteries Lymphadenopathy
Chest	Inspection Apex Chest expansion Percussion Lung field auscultation Heart sounds
Abdomen	Inspection Palpation Percussion
Neurological	Tone Power Reflexes (including plantars) Coordination
Skin	Rashes Needle marks
Peripheries	MedicAlert bracelet Pulses Joint inspection and palpation
Finish examination	Nutrition Height, weight (body mass index) if possible Urine output Assess hydration ECG Chest radiograph

Table 15.4 Secondary survey ('head-to-toe' examination)

This is a full history followed by a head-to-toe and front-to-back examination of the patient. It is particularly useful in patients who have been critically unwell or have sustained multiple injuries requiring immediate life-saving treatment. It ensures that less urgent problems are subsequently identified and managed appropriately.

15.3 Early warning score systems

Early Warning Score (EWS) systems provide a 'track-and-trigger' approach to efficiently identify and respond to patients who present with or develop acute illness. Six physiological parameters form the basis of the National EWS (NEWS) system produced by the Royal College of Physicians (**Figure 15.1**). The clinical response to NEWS triggers depend on the total score:

- **1–4:** low clinical risk
- **5–6** (or 3 in each parameter): medium clinical risk
- **>7:** high clinical risk

15.4 Adult advanced life support (Figure 15.2)

The ALS algorithm gives guidance as to how to manage a person in cardio–respiratory arrest. It is based upon the consensus between resuscitation experts from around the world. The underpinning concepts include:

- early recognition and call for help
- early cardiopulmonary resuscitation (CPR)
- early defibrillation
- post-resuscitation care

National early warning score (NEWS)

Physiological parameters	3	2	1	0	1	2	3
Respiration rate	≤8		9–11	12–20		21–24	≥25
Oxygen saturation	≤91	92–93	94–95	≥96			
Any supplemental oxygen		Yes		No			
Temperature	≤35.0		35.1–36.0	36.1–38.0	38.1–39.0	≥39.1	
Systolic BP	≤90	91–100	101–110	111–219			≥220
Heart rate	≤40		41–50	51–90	91–110	111–130	≥131
Level of consciousness				A			V, P, or U

Figure 15.1 National Early Warning Score (NEWS). With permission from: Royal College of Physicians, national early warning score (NEWS). Standardising the assessment of acute-illness severity in the NHS. London: Royal College of Physicians, 2012.

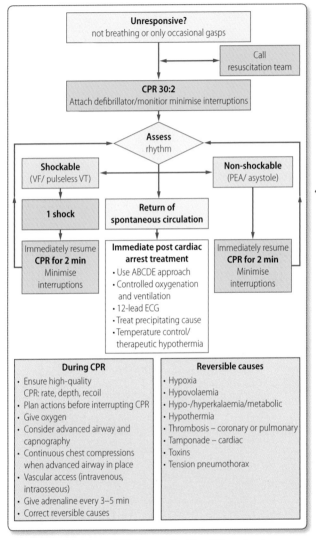

Figure 15.2 Adult Advanced Life Support algorithm. CPR, cardiopulmonary resuscitation. Reproduced with the kind permission of the Resuscitation Council (UK).

Index

Note: Page numbers in **bold** or *italic* refer to tables or figures respectively.

A

Abbreviated Mental Test (AMT) 191, **193**, 259, 301
ABC approach **279**, 283
ABCDE approach 305–10
Abdomen
  anatomy 103, *104*, *105*
  auscultation 115
  cardiovascular disease **64**
  common scars *114*
  critically ill patients **310**
  elderly patients 300
  gastrointestinal disease **110**, 111–12, 113–22
  genitourinary organs see Genitourinary system
  imaging investigations 125
  inspection 113–15, 154
  neonates **291**
  pain 106–7, **108**, 116–17, 133
  palpation 115–20, 154–5
  percussion 120–2
  pregnant women 154–5
  respiratory disease **91**
Abdominal aorta 73, 120
Abdominal aortic aneurysm **108**, 120
Abducens nerve (CN VI) **198**, 204–8
ABPI 80
Abused children 292
Accessory nerve (CN XI) **199**, 214
Active listening 3, 7
Activities of daily living 10, **11**
Addison's disease 265
Adolescents 277, **283**
  see also Paediatrics
Advanced life support algorithm 311, **313**
AEIOU TIPS mnemonic **308**
Affect 257
Air hunger 31
Airways, breathing, circulation (ABC) **279**, 283

Airways, breathing, circulation, disability, environment/exposure (ABCDE) 305–10
Alcohol use 12
Allergies 8–9
Alopecia 53
Ambulatory blood pressure monitoring 33
Amenorrhoea 145
Amniotic fluid volume 155
AMT see Abbreviated Mental Test (AMT)
Anal canal 104, 124
Ankle
  musculoskeletal examination **229**, *240–1*
  thyroid examination 270
Ankle–brachial pressure index (ABPI) 80
Anxiety 250
Aorta, palpation 73, 120
Aortic valves 57, *58*, **65**, *75*, **78**
Apex, palpation 96
Apex beat 71, *72*
APGAR score 289, **290**
Apnoea 31
Appendicitis **108**, **117**
Appendix *106*
Arm see Upper limb
Arterial bruits 80, 115
Ascites 111–12, 121–2
Asterixis 44, *45*, **169**
Asthma *100*
Atrioventricular valves
  anatomy 57
  apex beat 71
  cardiac cycle *58*
  cardiac pattern and diagnoses **65**
  heart sounds/murmurs **76**, 78
  surface markings *75*
Auditory function 210, *212*
Auditory hallucinations 257, 258
Auroscopy 49, *50*, 284
Auscultation 36–7
  see also specific systems
Autonomy 24, 25–6
AVPU scale **309**

B

Babinski's sign 183
Balanitis **132**
Barium studies 125
Basic activities of daily living (BADLs) 10, **11**
Beneficence 24
Biliary colic **108**
Bimanual pelvic examination 151–2
Bladder *see* Urinary bladder
Blood
    abnormal bleeding in women 145
    coughed up (haemoptysis) 90–1
    in stools 109
    in urine (haematuria) 129
    vomiting (haematemesis) 109
Blood oxygen saturation *see* Oxygen
    saturation
Blood pressure 60, 63
    ankle–brachial pressure index 80
    elderly patients 298
    measurement 32–3, **34**, 80
    National Early Warning Score **312**
    ophthalmological investigations 216
    paediatric patients 283
Blood tests
    cardiovascular disease 82
    dementia 301
    endocrine disease 272
    musculoskeletal disease 245
    psychiatric assessment 260
    respiratory disease 101
    sexually transmitted infections 135
Blumberg's sign **117**
Body mass index (BMI) 38–9
Body surface area (BSA) 39, 276
Bones **224**
Borborygmi 105, 115
Bouchard's nodes **228**, **230**
Boutonnière's deformity **228**, **230**
Bowel sounds 105, 115
Bradycardia 63
Bragard's test 235, *244*
Brain
    anatomy 159–60
    visual fields *200*
    see also Neurological system
Breast 137, *138*, 139–45, **158**, **266**, **303**
    examination 142–5, **158**
Breast tissue (gynaecomastia) 111, **266**
Breath smells 113
Breath sounds, reduced 92

Breathing
    ABC approach **279**, 283
    ABCDE approach **305**, 307
    advanced life support **313**
    bronchial 92
    cardiac pathology 61–2
    paediatric patients 276, **279**, 281,
        283, **290**
    patterns 30–1, 38
    physiology 86–7
Breathlessness 30, 61–2, 89–90
Broca's aphasia **192**
Bronchial breathing 92
Bronchial tree 85
Bronchoscopy 101
Brudzinski's test 189
Bruising 113
Bruits, arterial 80, 115
BSA *see* Body surface area (BSA)

C

CAGE questionnaire 12
Candida albicans 147
Capacity 25
Capillary refill time 33–4, 284
Carbon dioxide 87
Cardiac subjects *see* Heart
Cardiogenic shock 40
Cardiopulmonary resuscitation 25, 311,
    313
Cardiovascular system 57–83
    ABC approach **279**, 283
    ABCDE approach **305**, 307–8
    anatomy 57–9
    auscultation 73–8, *79*, 80, **285**
    cardiac patterns **65–6**
    causes of fever **31**
    critically ill patients **305**, 307–8, 311,
        313
    elderly patients 293, 297–8, 299
    examination 65–83, **83**
    general inspection 66, 79
    history taking **15**, **61**
    investigations 82
    jugular venous pressure 59, **65**,
        66–9, 94
    paediatric patients 276, **279**, **280**,
    281–2, 283, **285**
    palpation 71–3, 79–80, 81, **285**
    percussion 73, **285**

physiology *58*, 59–60
pulse assessment 30, **34**, 69–70, *74*, 80
signs of dehydration/shock **40**
signs of disease **41**, **44**, 63–5, **64**
symptoms of disease 60–3
Carotid arterial pressure **69**
Carotid ultrasonography 82
Carpal tunnel assessment 235–8
Case presentation 20, *21*
Central nervous system 159–62
Cerebellum 162, 172, 189
Cerebrospinal fluid analysis 194
Cervix of uterus *138*, *139*
abnormal bleeding 145
colposcopy 157
examination 148–51
smear and swabs 150, 157
Chest
cardiovascular examination **64**, **65**, 71–2, 73–8
critically ill patients **310**
elderly patients **303**
gastrointestinal disease **110**
inspection 95
musculoskeletal disease **224**
neonates **291**
pain 60–1, **62**
percussion *36*, 91–2, 97, *99*
radiographs 82, 101, 125
respiratory disease 91–3
respiratory examination 95, 97–9
surface anatomy *86*
Cheyne–Stokes respiration 30
Child abuse 292
Chlamydia infection 147
Cholangiopancreatography 126
Cholecystitis **117**
Circulation
ABC approach **279**, 283
ABCDE approach **305**, 307–8
see also Cardiovascular system
Claudication 63
Clock drawing 191
Clonus 174
Clubbing 42, *43*, **44**, 267
CNs *see* Cranial nerves (CNs)
Cochlear function **198**, 210, *212*
Codes of practice 22–4
Cognitive function 191–4, 259, 297–8, 301
Collateral ligament stability 240–1, *246*

Colonoscopy 126
Colour
APGAR score **290**
general inspection 38
see also Cyanosis; Jaundice
Colposcopy 157
Compulsions 250–1
Computed tomography 194, 246
Confidentiality 13, 25
Congestive heart failure 59
Consciousness
ABCDE approach 308–9
AVPU scale **309**
delirium 251
Glasgow Coma Scale **309**
level of 191
National Early Warning Score **312**
paediatric patients 284, **309**
sudden loss of (syncope) 63, 164
Consent 25, 28, 35
Consolidation, lung *100*
Constipation 109, 300
Consultations 1
active listening 3, 7
adolescents 277
clinical examination *see* Clinical examination
differential diagnosis 17–19
documenting 19–20
elderly patients 295
end of 19
environment for 4
history taking 1, **2**, 3–17
psychiatric 251
question techniques 1–3, 7, 16
Coordination 187–9
Coronary angiography 82
Corrigan's sign **65**
Cough 88–9
Crackles (crepitations) 64–5, 78, 92, 299–300
Cranial nerves (CNs)
anatomy 197–9
examination 202–14, **217–18**
eye movements **197**, **198**, *201*, 204–5
Cremasteric reflex 133–4
Crepitations *see* Crackles
Critically ill patients 305–13
advanced life support 311, **313**
early warning score 311, **312**

examination 305–13
   primary survey 305–10
   secondary survey 310–11
Cruciate ligaments 241–2, *247*
Cyanosis 38, 94

D

Deafness 210, *212*, 295
Decision-making ethics 22, 24, 25–6
Deep tendon reflexes *see* Reflexes
Deep vein thrombosis (DVT) 80
Dehydration 39, **40**, 281
Delirium 191, **193**, 194, 251, 297
DELIRIUM mnemonic 251
Dementia 191, **193**, 194, 296–7, 301–2
Depression 249
Dermatomes 160, *161*, 184
Development assessment 286–9
DH *see* Drug history (DH)
Diabetes 264, 270–1, 272
Diarrhoea 109
Differential diagnosis 17–19
Digital rectal examination 122–5, 300
Disability, ABCDE approach **305**, 308–9
Distributive shock 40
DNA SORAN mnemonic 1, **2**
Doctor–patient relationship 1, 3
Documentation 19–20
Draw test 241–2, *247*
Dropped finger **228**, **230**
Drug history (DH) **2**, 4, 7–8
   breast disease **141**
   cardiovascular disease **61**
   elderly patients **294**
   endocrine disease **265**
   gastrointestinal disease **107**
   gynaecological disease **146**
   musculoskeletal disease **220**
   neurological disease **163**
   paediatric patients 277, **278**
   pregnant women **153**
   psychiatric assessment 253–4
   respiratory disease **88**
Drug use, illicit 13
Dual-energy X-ray absorptiometry (DEXA) 247
Dupuytren's contracture 42
Durkan's compression 238
Durosier's sign **66**
DVT *see* Deep vein thrombosis (DVT)
Dysarthria **192**

Dysdiadochokinesia 187
Dysfluency **192**
Dyspareunia 145
Dysphagia 107–9
Dysphasia **192**
Dysphasia **192**
Dysphonia **192**
Dyspnoea *see* Breathlessness
Dysuria 129

E

Ear
   CN VIII function 210–12, *213*
   elderly patients 295, 299
   general inspection 49, *50*
   paediatric patients 284, 286
Early warning score (EWS) 311, **312**
EBM *see* Evidence-based medicine (EBM)
Echocardiography 82
Ectopic pregnancy **108**
Elbow examination **228**, *236*
Elderly patients 293–304
   examination 297–302, **303**
   functional age 293
   history taking 294–5
   multidisciplinary teams 302
   physiological changes 293–4
   symptoms 295–7
Electrocardiography 82
Electroencephalography 194
Electromyography 194
Emotional state 38, 257
Endocrine system 261–73
   anatomy 261, *262*
   diabetes 264, 270–1, 272
   history taking 262, **265**
   investigations 272
   physiology 261–2, *263*
   signs of disease **41**, 266–7
   symptoms of disease 264–6
   thyroid examination 267–70, **273**
Endoscopy, gastrointestinal 125–6
Epididymis **132**, 133, *134*
Epispadias 133
Erectile dysfunction 130
Erythema, palmar 42
Ethicolegal considerations 22–6
Evidence-based medicine (EBM) 20–2, *23*
Exposure
   ABCDE approach **305**, 309–10
   for examination 29, 112

Eye
  anatomy *201*
  cardiovascular disease **64**, 79
  colour vision 204
  dehydration **40**
  elderly patients 299, **303**
  endocrine disease **266**, 268
  examination 214–16
  gastrointestinal disease **110**, 112–13
  general inspection **37**
  innervation **197–8**, 199, *200*
  investigations 216–17
  movements **197**, **198**, *201*, 204–5
  musculoskeletal disease **224**
  neonates 291
  neurological disease **166**
  ophthalmoscopy 204, *205–6*
  pupil 94, **197**, *201*, 205–8
  respiratory disease 94
  visual acuity 202, 214, 295
  visual fields *200*, 202–14, 217, 267
  visual symptoms 199–201

F

Face
  cardiovascular disease **64**
  cutaneous innervation **198**, *209*
  elderly patients 299, **303**
  endocrine disease **266**, **268**
  facial nerve examination **198**, 210, *211*
  gastrointestinal disease **110**, 111
  general inspection **37**, 48
  musculoskeletal disease **224**
  neurological disease **166**
  respiratory disease **91**
  veins of *68*
Facial nerve (CN VII) **198**, 210, *211*
Fainting 63, 164
Faith history 11–12
Fallopian tubes, palpation 152
Falls, elderly patients 296, 298
Family history (FH) **2**, 4, 9
  breast disease **141**
  cardiovascular disease **61**
  endocrine disease **265**
  gastrointestinal disease **107**
  gynaecological disease **146**
  musculoskeletal disease **220**
  neurological disease **163**

  paediatric patients **278**, 279
  pregnant women **153**
  psychiatric assessment 254
  respiratory disease **88**
Family trees *9*
Female reproductive system 137–58
  anatomy 127, 137–9
  breast 137, *138*, 139–45, **158**
  examination summary **158**
  gynaecology 139, **140**, 143, 145–52, **158**
  history taking 137, 139–40, **141**, 143
  investigations 157
  obstetric examination 152–7, **158**
  physiology 139
Femoral hernias **132**, 134, 135
Femoral nerve stretch test 235, *245*
Fetor hepaticus 113
Fetuses, obstetrics 154–7
Fever 31–2
  elderly patients 297
  paediatric patients 280, 281, 283
FH *see* Family history (FH)
Fibrosis, lung *100*
Finger nails *see* Nails
Finger rub test, hearing 210
Fits (seizures) 164–5, 266
Flap 44
  see also Tremor
Fluid thrills 122
Fluorescein, topical 217
Fluorescein angiography 217
Foot **37**, 52, 181–3, **229**
Fundus fluorescein angiography 217

G

Gait 169–72
  elderly patients 300
  GALS assessment 223–4, 225, **285**
Gallbladder 103, *105*, 117
GALS assessment 223–7, **285**
Gas exchange, lungs 87
Gastrointestinal system 103–26
  anatomy 103–4, *105–6*
  auscultation 115
  causes of chest pain *62*
  causes of fever *31*
  digital rectal examination 122–5, 300
  elderly patients 293, 300
  examination 112–26, **126**
  history taking **15**, **107**

inspection 112–15, **285**
investigations 125–6
paediatric patients **280**, **285**
palpation 115–20, **285**
percussion 120–2
physiology 105
proctoscopy 124
prostate examination 123, 125
signs of disease **41**, **44**, 110–12
symptoms of disease 106–10
Genetic disorders 287–9
family trees *9*
see also Family history
Genitourinary system
anatomy 127, *128*, 137–9
cardiovascular disease **64**, 73
causes of fever **31**
endocrine disease **266**
examination summary **135**, **158**
female 127, 137–9, 145–57, **158**
gastrointestinal disease **110**
history taking **15**, **129**, 130–1, 143, **146**
investigations 135, 157
male 127–35
Get-up-and-go test 300, 301
Glasgow Coma Scale **309**
Glossopharyngeal nerve (CN IX) **198**, 213–14
Glucose test, ABCDE approach 309
Glycaemic control 262, *264*, 266
Goitre **266**, 267, 268
Goniometers 233
Gonioscopy 217
Gonorrhoea 147
Graphaesthesia 187
Graves' disease 267
Groin lumps **132**
Growth, paediatric patients 286
Gunstock deformity **230**
Gynaecology 139, **140**, 143, 145–52, **158**
examination 147–52, **158**
Gynaecomastia 111, **266**

H

Haematemesis 109
Haematuria 129
Haemoptysis 90–1
Hair 53, 265, 267
Hallpike's manoeuvre 212, *213*
Hallucinations 257, 258

Hand
cardiovascular disease **41**, **44**, 64
deformities 230
endocrine disease **41**, 266, 267, 268
gastrointestinal disease **41**, **44**, 110, 113
general inspection **37**, 41–5, **55**
hand hygiene 28
movement coordination tests 187–9
musculoskeletal disease **41**, **224**, 225
musculoskeletal examination 227, **228**, **230**, *231*, *237*–8
neonates **291**
osteoarthritis **222**
respiratory disease **41**, **44**, **91**
rheumatoid arthritis **222**
Head
critically ill patients **310**
elderly patients 299, **303**
neonates **291**
Headache 162–3
Hearing **198**, 210, *212*
development 287, **288**–9
elderly patients 295, 299
Heart
advanced life support algorithm **313**
anatomy 57
auscultation 73–8, *79*
cardiac cycle *58*, 59
cardiac output 59
cardiac patterns and diagnoses **65**–6
chest wall percussion 73
elderly patients 298, 299
failure 59, 62, **65**
fetal 157
investigations 82
jugular venous pressure **65**, 66–7
murmurs **65**–6, 72, 76–8, 281–2, 299
National Early Warning Score **312**
paediatric patients **280**, 281–2
palpation 71–3
signs of disease 63–5
sounds (S1/S2/extra) 57, **65**, 66, 73–5, **76**
symptoms of disease 60–3
Heaves 71, *72*
Heberden's nodes **230**
Height, children 286, **287**
Hepatojugular reflex 67
Hepatomegaly 117, *118*, 120–1

Hernias **132**, 133, 134, 135
Hip examination **229**, **230**, 238–9
History of presenting complaint (HPC) **2**, 4, 5–6
   psychiatric assessment 252, **253**
History taking 1, **2**, 3–17
   allergies 8–9
   drug history **2**, 7–8
   family history **2**, 9
   history of presenting complaint **2**, 5–6
   ICEs 14
   immunisation history 9
   past medical history **2**, 6–7
   past surgical history **2**, 6–7
   pitfalls 15–16
   presenting complaint 4–5
   social history **2**, 10–14
   summarising 17
   systems review 14, **15**
   see also specific systems
HIV/AIDS 40
Horner's syndrome 94, **207**
Hydration 39–40, 281
Hydrocele 133
Hyperbilirubinaemia 111
Hyperglycaemia 266, 309
Hyperkyphosis **230**
Hyperpyrexia 32
Hypertension 33, 63
Hyperthyroidism *268*, 270
Hypertonia 165–6
Hypoglossal nerve (CN XII) **199**, 214
Hypoglycaemia 266, 309
Hypomania 249
Hypospadias 133
Hypotension 33, 63, 283, 298
Hypothalamopituitary axis (HPA) 261, *263*
Hypothermia 31, 32
Hypothyroidism *268*, 270
Hypovolaemic shock 40

I

IADLs *see* Instrumental activities of daily living (IADLs)
Iatrogenic problems 297
Ideas, concerns and effects or expectations (ICEs) 14
Ileus 115
Illusions 257

Immobility 296
Immunisation history 9
Incontinence 145, 296, 300
Inguinal region
   anatomy 127, *128*
   hernias **132**, 134, 135
   inspection 134
Inherited disease 287–9
   family trees 9
   see also Family history
Insight 258
Instability 296
Instrumental activities of daily living (IADLs) 10, **11**
Interferon gamma release assay 101
Intermenstrual bleeding (IMB) 145
Investigations 18–19
   see also specific systems
Ischaemic heart disease 60–1

J

JADE CAT MARCH mnemonic **7**
Janeway's lesions 42
Jaundice 111
Jaw jerk 208
Joints
   active movement **228**, **229**, 233, *234–43*
   effusions 223, 240
   GALS assessment 225, 226
   inspection 227, **228–9**
   investigations 245, 246
   loss of function 221–2
   osteoarthritis 221, **222**
   pain 219–20, *221*, 222–3, 233
   palpation 227–31
   passive movement **228**, **229**, 233, 235
   position sense 184, *185*
   range of movement 232–3, *234–43*
   rheumatoid arthritis 221, **222**
   special tests **228**, **229**, 235–42, *244–7*
   stability 233
   stiffness 221
   swelling 222–3
   types 219
Jugular venous pressure (JVP) 59, **65**, 66–9, 94
Justice 24

K

Kayser–Fleischer rings 112–13
Kernig's sign 189
Ketosis 113
Kidney, palpation **118**, 119
Knee examination **229**, 240–2, *246*
Koilonychia 42, **55**
Korotkoff's sounds 33
Kussmaul's respiration 30–1
Kwashiorkor 286, **287**
Kyphosis *226*, **228**, **230**, 299

L

Labour 155–7, 277
Lachman's test 242, *247*
Language abnormalities **166**, 191, **192**
Language development 287, **288–9**
Large intestine 103, *105–6*, **108**, 126
Laseque's test *244*
Leg *see* Lower limb
Legal concepts 22–6
Leukonychia 42, **55**
Libido 130
Listening 3, 7
Lithotomy position 147, *148*
Liver
    anatomy 103, *105*
    investigations 125
    palpation 73, 117, **118**, *119*
    percussion 120–1
Lobectomy, lung *100*
Lordosis *22*, **228**, **230**
Lower limb
    coordination 189, *190*
    GALS assessment (Legs) 223–4, 226,
        285
    general inspection **37**, 52
    meningism tests 189
    muscle tone *173*, 174
    musculoskeletal examination **229**,
        232, 233, 238–42, *246–7*
    neonates **291**
    peripheral vascular system 57–9, 63,
        64, 65, 79–82
    power *177–9*, 179
    reflexes 181–3
    respiratory disease **91**
Lumps
    breast 140–1, 143–5
    groin **132**

lymph node **47**, **132**
    scrotal **132**, 133
Lung
    anatomy 85, *86*
    bronchoscopy 101
    CT pulmonary angiography 101
    elderly patients **303**
    function tests 101
    gas exchange 87
    main pathologies *100*
    signs of disease 91–3
    symptoms of disease 94
    vocal resonance 99
Lymph nodes 45–7, *48*, 97

M

Magnetic resonance imaging 194, 216, 247
Mallet finger **228**, **230**
Malnutrition 39, 286, **287**
Management 18
Mania 249
Marasmus 286, **287**
Mastalgia 141
McBurney's point **117**
McMurray's test 242
Median nerve compression 235–8
Medical history *see* Past medical history
    (PMH)
Medical notes 19–20
Medication history *see* Drug history
Melaena 109
Memory 191, **193**, 296–7, 301
Meningism 189
Meniscal tears 242
Menstruation
    abnormal bleeding 145
    menstrual cycle 139, **140**
    menstrual history 143
Mental state assessment 38, **193**, 194,
    256–9, 301
Mental State Examination (MSE) 256–9
Micturition 129–30
Mini-mental state examination (MMSE)
    193, 194, 301
Mistreated children 292
Mitral valve *see* Atrioventricular valves
Mood 257
Motor development 286–7, **288–9**
Motor functions, CNs **198**, 208, 210, 213
Motor pathways 159–60

Motor power **167**, 174–9, *180*

Mouth
    cardiovascular disease **64**
    elderly patients 299, **303**
    gastrointestinal disease **110**, 111,
        113
    general inspection **37**, 48–9
    neonates **291**
    see also Throat

Movement abnormalities **169**, 174
    CN XII **214**
    eye **204–5**
    joint examination 232–3, *234–43*
    see also Tremor

Multidisciplinary teams 301

Murphy's sign **117**

Muscle power **167**, 174–9, *180*

Muscle tone 165–6, **167**, 172–4, **290**

Musculoskeletal system 219–48
    anatomy 219
    causes of chest pain **62**
    elderly patients 293, 301, **303**
    examination 223–43, **248**
    GALS assessment 223–7, **285**
    history taking **15**, 219, **220**, 224
    investigations 243–7
    joint examination 227–43, **248**
    paediatric patients **280**, **285**
    red flags 221
    signs of disease **41**, 222–3, **224**
    symptoms of disease 219–22

N

Nails
    general inspection **41**, 42, *43*, **44**, 53,
        55
    thyroid disease 267

National EWS (NEWS) system 311, **312**

Nausea 109

Neck
    cardiovascular disease **64**
    critically ill patients **310**
    deformities **230**
    elderly patients **303**
    gastrointestinal disease **110**
    general inspection **37**, 45–7, *48*
    goitre **266**, 267, 268
    meningism 189
    musculoskeletal disease **224**

    musculoskeletal examination **228**,
        230, 233, *242*
    neonates **291**
    respiratory disease **91**
    veins of *68*

Neonates 275, 289–92

Nerve conduction studies 194, 247

Neurological system 159–95
    abbreviated assessment 168, **193**
    ABCDE approach 309–10
    anatomy 159–62
    causes of fever **31**
    cerebellar function 172, 189
    coordination 187–9
    critically ill patients **310**
    dehydration/shock **40**
    elderly patients 293, 300, 301, **303**
    examination equipment *168*
    examination 166–95, **195**
    gait 169–72, 300
    general inspection 168–9, **285**
    higher mental function 191–4, 301
    history taking **15**, 162–3, 164–5
    investigations 194
    meningism tests 189
    paediatric patients **280**, **285**, 290,
        309
    physiology 162
    positioning the patient 167
    power **167**, 174–9, *180*
    reflexes 162, **166**, **167**, 181–3
    sensation **166**, 183–7
    signs of disease **41**, 165–6
    symptoms of disease 162–5
    tone 165–6, **167**, 172–4, **290**
    see also Cranial nerves; Ophthalmology;
        Psychiatric assessment

NEWS system 311, **312**

Nipples 142, 143

Nocturia 129

Nocturnal dyspnoea 30, 62

Non-maleficence 24

Nose 49–50, *51*, **291**

Note making 19–20

Nutrition
    clinical assessment 38–9
    elderly patients 298
    history taking 13–14, **278**
    paediatric patients 278, 286, **287**

Nystagmus 204–5

O

Observations *see* Vital signs
Obsessions 250
Obstetric examination 152–7, **158**
Obstructive sleep apnoea 31
Oculomotor nerve (CN III) **197**, 204–8
Odynophagia 107–9
Oedema 59, 62, 64–5, 73
Olfactory nerve (CN I) **197**
OPERATES+ mnemonic **2**, **5**, **253**
Ophthalmology
  cardiovascular examination 79
  cranial nerve examinations 202–8
  eye anatomy 201
  eye innervation **197**, 199, *200*
  investigations 216–17
  visual symptoms 199–201
  visual system examination 202–4, 214–16
Ophthalmoscopy 204, *205–6*
Optic disc 204, *206*
Optic nerve (CN II) **197**, 199, 202–4, 208
Optic tract 199, *200*
Optical coherence tomography 217
Orchitis **132**
Orthopnoea 61–2
Orthostatic hypotension 33, 298
Osler's nodes 42
Osteoarthritis 221, **222**
Otoscopes 49, *50*, *51*, 284
Ovaries 152
Oxygen
  advanced life support **313**
  central cyanosis 94
  delivery devices 95
  partial pressure 34
  respiration 87
  supplemental 94, 95, 307, **312**, **313**
Oxygen saturation (pulse oximetry) 34
  elderly patients 298
  National Early Warning Score **312**
  paediatric patients **283**

P

Paediatrics 275–92
  age definitions 275
  anatomy 275, *276*
  AVPU scale **309**
  child mistreatment 292
  clinical environment 275
  development assessment 286–9
  examining children 282–6
  examining neonates 289–92
  history taking 277–9, 287
  key symptoms 280
  physiology 276
  red flags 277–9, **279**
Paget's disease 143
Pain history **2**, 5, **6**
Pain sensation 185–6
Palms 42
Palpation 35
  lymph nodes 46–7, 97
  see also specific systems
Palpitations 62–3
Pancreas
  abdominal pain **108**
  anatomy 103, *105*
  glycaemic control 262
  investigations 125, 126
Parotid glands 48
Paroxysmal nocturnal dyspnoea 30
Past medical history (PMH) **2**, 4, 6–7
  breast disease **141**
  cardiovascular disease **61**
  elderly patients **294**
  endocrine disease **265**
  gastrointestinal disease **107**
  genitourinary disease **129**, 143, **146**
  musculoskeletal disease **220**
  neurological disease **163**
  paediatric patients **278**
  pregnant women **153**
  psychiatric assessment 253
  respiratory disease **88**
Past surgical history (PSH) **2**, 4, 6–7
  cardiovascular disease **61**
  elderly patients **294**
  gastrointestinal disease **107**
  musculoskeletal disease **220**
  neurological disease **163**
  pregnant women **153**
  psychiatric assessment 253
  respiratory disease **88**
Patent ductus arteriosus (PDA) 281
PC *see* Presenting complaint (PC)
PCB *see* Postcoital bleeding (PCB)
Pelvic examination 147, 150–2
Pelvic pain 145
Pelvis, fetal engagement 155
Penis **132**, 133

Peptic ulcers **108**
Perceptions, abnormal 257–8
Percussion 35–6
    see also specific systems
Peripheral oedema 59, 65, 73
Peripheral vascular system 57–9
    auscultation 80
    elderly patients 299
    inspection 79
    mid-calf diameter 82
    palpation 79–80, 81
    signs of disease **64**, 65
    symptoms of disease 63
Peristalsis 105
Peritoneum 103, **108**, **117**
Personal history 254, **255**
Phalen's test 235
Phimosis **132**, 133
Phobias 250
Pituitary tumours 267
Plantar reflex 181–3
Pleural effusion *100*
PMH *see* Past medical history (PMH)
Pneumonectomy *100*
Pneumothorax *100*
Polydipsia 264, 266
Polyuria 264, 266
Position sense 172, 184, *185*
Positioning of patients 28, 112, 142–3, 147, 167
    paediatric 284
Postcoital bleeding (PCB) 145
Postural hypotension 33, 298
Power (muscle) **167**, 174–9, *180*
Prayer signs 225, 235
Pregnancy
    ectopic **108**
    obstetrics 152–7, **158**
    paediatric history taking 277
Presentation of cases 20, *21*
Presenting complaint (PC) **2**, 4–5
    breast **141**
    cardiovascular **61**
    elderly patients **294**
    endocrine **265**
    gastrointestinal **107**
    genitourinary **129**, **146**
    history of **2**, 4, 5–6, 252, **253**
    musculoskeletal **220**
    neurological **163**
    obstetric **153**

paediatric patients **278**
    psychiatric assessment 252, **253**
    respiratory **88**
Privacy 28
Probity 26
Pronator drift 179
Proprioception 172
Prostate
    abdominal pain **108**
    anatomy 127
    examination 123, 125
    investigations 135
    micturition problems 129–30
Proximal myopathy 267–8
Pruritus 113
Pseudohallucinations 258
PSH *see* Past surgical history (PSH)
Psychiatric assessment 249–60
    elderly patients 301
    higher mental function 259
    history taking 251–6
    investigations 259–60
    Mental State Examination 256–9
    physical examination 259
    summary **260**
    symptoms 249–51
Psychotic symptoms 250
Pulmonary oedema 59, 62, 64–5
Pulmonary valve 57, *58*, 75, **78**
Pulse oximetry *see* Oxygen saturation
Pulse(s)
    assessment 30, **34**, 69–70, *74*, 80
    cardiovascular disease 63, **64**, **70**
    elderly patients 297–8
    endocrine disease **268**
    paediatric patients **283**, **290**
Pupil 94, **197**, *201*, 205–8
Pyrexia 31, 32
Pyrogens 32

Q

Question types 1–3, 7, 16
Quincke's sign **65**

R

Radiography 82, 101, 125, 245
Record keeping 19–20
Rectum
    anatomy 103, 104, *105*, *106*
    bleeding 109

digital examination 122–5, 300
proctoscopy 124
Reflex irritability, neonates **290**
Reflexes 162, **166**, **167**, 181–3, 270
Relative afferent pupillary defect (RAPD) 208
Religion, faith history 10–11
Renal colic **108**
Resistance testing 174, *175–9*
Respiration
ABC approach **279**, 283
ABCDE approach **305**, 307
advanced life support **313**
breathlessness 30, 61–2, 89–90
cardiac pathology 61–2
National Early Warning Score **312**
paediatric patients 276, **279**, 281, **290**
patterns of 30–1, 38
physiology 86–7
Respiratory failure 87
Respiratory rate 30–1, **34**
elderly patients 298
National Early Warning Score **312**
paediatric patients 283
Respiratory system 85–102
anatomy 85, *86*
auscultation 97–9, **285**
cardiovascular disease 61–2, 64–5
causes of fever **31**
chest percussion *36*, 91–2, 97, *99*, **285**
critically ill patients **305**, 307, 311,
312, **313**
elderly patients 293, 298, 299–300,
303
examination 93–102, **102**
history taking **15**, 87, **88**
inspection 93–5, **285**
investigations 101
main lung pathologies *100*
paediatric patients **279**, **280**, 281,
283, **285**, **290**
palpation 95–7, **285**
physiology 86–7
signs of disease **41**, **44**, 91–3
symptoms of disease 88–91
upper respiratory tract *see* Mouth; Nose
Resuscitation 25, 311, **313**
Retching 109
Reticular activating system 162
Rheumatoid arthritis 221, **222**
Rigidity 165, 166

Rigor 32
Rinne's test 210, *212*
Risk assessment, psychiatric 258
Romberg's test 172
Rovsing's sign **117**
Rubs 92–3

S

Sackett's five steps for EBM 22, *23*
SAD PERSONS mnemonic 258–9
Scapula **230**
Schizophrenia 250
Schober's test 235
Sciatic nerve stretch test 235, *244*
Scoliosis *226*, **228**, **230**
Scratch marks 113
Scrotum *128*, **132**, 133, 135
Seizures 164–5, 266
Sensory examination **166**, 183–7
Sensory functions, CNs **198**, 209, 210,
213–14
Sensory pathways 160, *161*, 184
Sexual function 130
Sexual history 130–1
Sexual intercourse 145
Sexually transmitted infections (STIs) 130,
131, **132**, 135, 147, 150
SH *see* Social history (SH)
Shock 39–40
Shortness of breath (SOB) *see* Breathlessness
Shoulder examination **228**, **230**, *234*
Skeletal system 219
see also Musculoskeletal system
Skin
breast tumours 143
critically ill patients **310**
elderly patients 298–9, **303**
endocrine disease 265, **266**, 267, **268**
gastrointestinal disease **110**
general assessment **37**, 38, **40**, 52–3
graphaesthesia 187
lesion types *54*
musculoskeletal disease **224**
pregnancy changes 154
Sleep apnoea 31
Small intestine 103, *106*, 125–6
Smell
of breath 113
sense of **197**, 202
Smoking 11

SOB (shortness of breath) *see* Breathlessness
Social development 287, **288–9**
Social history (SH) **2**, 4, 10–14
    breast disease **141**
    cardiovascular disease **61**
    elderly patients **294**
    endocrine disease **265**
    gastrointestinal disease **107**
    genitourinary disease **129**, 130–1, **146**
    musculoskeletal disease **220**
    neurological disease **163**
    paediatric patients **278**
    pregnant women **153**
    psychiatric assessment 254
    respiratory disease **88**
SOCRATES mnemonic **2**, 5, **6**
Spasticity 165
Speculum examinations 148–50, 152, 157
Speech **166**, 191, **192**, 256
Spider naevi 113
Spinal cord 160, *161*, 184
Spinal tap 194
Spine
    deformities **230**
    elderly patients 299
    GALS assessment 223–4, 226–7, **285**
    musculoskeletal disease **224**
    musculoskeletal examination **228**,
        230, 233, 235, *243–5*
Spiritual history 10–11
Spleen *105–6*, 118, *119*, 120, 121
Splenomegaly 118
Splinter haemorrhages 42, **55**
Sputum 90, 101
Squint 215–16
SSS CCC FFF TTT mnemonic 45, **47**
Starling's law 59
Stenosing tenosynovitis *see* Trigger finger
Stereognosis 186
Stethoscopes 36–7, 97
STIs *see* Sexually transmitted infections (STIs)
Stomach 103, *105*
Stools 109, 125
Strabismus 215–16
Straight leg raise 235, *244*
Stretch reflexes *see* Reflexes
Stridor 93
Suicidal assessment 258–9
Surgical history *see* Past surgical history (PSH)
Swallowing, problems with 107–9
Swan-neck deformity **228**, **230**

Symphyseal–fundal height 154, *155*
Syncope 63, 164
Systemic vascular resistance (SVR) 59–60

T

Tachycardia 63
Tactile vocal fremitus 97
Taste sense **198**
Teeth 49
Temperature 31–2, **34**
    elderly patients 297
    National Early Warning Score **312**
    paediatric patients 280, 281, 283
Temperature sensation 185–6
Tendon reflexes *see* Reflexes
Testicles
    anatomy 127, *128*
    carcinoma **132**, 133
    cremasteric reflex 133–4
    pain 130, **132**
    palpation 133, *134*
    signs of disease **132**
    torsion **132**, 133
    ultrasound 135
Thirst, polydipsia 264, 266
Thomas's test 239
Thoughts 257
Thrills 72, 122, 281
Throat 50, *51*, 284–5, 286
Thudicum speculum *51*
Thyroid
    anatomy 261, *262*
    auscultation 270
    examination **41**, 267–70, **273**
    goitre **266**, 267, 268
    investigations 272
    palpation 268–9
    regulation 261, *263*
Thyroid acropachy 267
Tinel's sign 238
Toe movements *241*
Toe nails *see* Nails
Tone (muscle) 165–6, **167**, 172–4, **290**
Tongue
    general inspection 48–9, 94
    innervation **198**, **199**, 210, 214
Tonometry 217
Tophi 43
Torticollis **228**, **230**
Touch sensation 184, 186, 187
Trachea 85, *86*, 95–6

Tremor 44, *45*, 165, **169**, 267
Trendelenburg's test (hip) 239–40
Trendelenburg's test (veins) 81
Trichomonas vaginalis 147
Tricuspid valve *see* Atrioventricular valves
Trigeminal nerve (CN V) **198**, 208–9
Trigger finger **228**, **230**
Trochlear nerve (CN IV) **197**, 204–8
Tympanic membrane 49, *50*, 284

U

Ulcers
　genital **132**
　peptic **108**
Ultrasound 82, 125, 132, 216, 272
Undernutrition 39, 286, **287**
Upper limb
　active movements 233
　coordination 187–9
　deformities **230**
　endocrine disease 267
　GALS assessment (Arms) 223–4,
　　225–6, **285**
　joint examination **228**, **230**, 232–3, *234*,
　　235–8
　muscle tone 172, *173*
　neonates 291
　power *175–6*, 179
　reflexes 181, *182*
　see also Hand
Uraemic fetor 113
Urethra (female) 127, *138*
Urethra (male) 127, 130, *133*
Urinary bladder
　abdominal pain **108**
　palpation 119
　symptoms of disease 130
Urinary tract, anatomy 127
Urine
　blood in (haematuria) 129
　incontinence of 145, 296
　investigations 125, 135
　micturition problems 129–30
　polyuria 264, 266
Urine tests
　endocrine disease 272
　genitourinary assessment 157
　musculoskeletal disease 245
　psychiatric assessment 260
Uterus 137–9, 145, 151–2, 154–5, *156*

V

Vagina 137–9, 147, 148–52, 155–7
Vaginosis, bacterial 147
Vagus nerve (CN X) **198**, 213–14
Valgus deformities 227
Values, patient 21
Varicocele **132**, 133
Varicose veins 81
Varus deformities 227, **230**
Vestibular function **198**, 212, *213*
Vestibulocochlear nerve (CN VIII) **198**,
　210–12, *213*
Vibration sensation 184–5, *186*
Virus serology 101
Vision development 287, **288–9**
Visual acuity 202, 214, 295
Visual fields *200*, 202–4, 214, 217, 267
Visual symptoms 199–201
Visual system examination 214–16
Visual tract 199, *200*
Vital signs 29–34
　cardiovascular disease 63, **64**, 80
　dehydration/shock **40**
　elderly patients 297–8
　musculoskeletal disease **224**
　National Early Warning Score **312**
　paediatric patients 280, 283, **287**,
　　291
　respiratory disease **91**
VITAMIN CDE mnemonic 17
Vocal fremitus 97, 99
Vocal resonance 97–9
Vomiting 109

W

Weakness 165, 174–9, *180*
Weber's test 210, *212*
Weight, children 276, 286, **287**
Weight change 109–10, 264–5, **268**
Wernicke's aphasia **192**
Wheeze 93
Whisper test, hearing 210
Whispering pectoriloquy e99
Wrist deformities **230**
Wrist examination **228**, **230**, *231*, 235–8

X

Xanthomas 43
　xanthelasma 113